A TIMEKEEPER'S GUIDE
TO WEIGHT LOSS

LIVING AN INTERMITTENT FASTING LIFESTYLE, WATCHING WHEN YOU EAT, NOT WHAT YOU EAT

DONNA DUBE, MS, RN

outskirts
press

Outskirts Press, Inc.
http://www.outskirtspress.com

Paperback ISBN: 978-1-9772-0610-7

Outskirts Press and the "OP" logo are trademarks belonging to Outskirts Press, Inc.

PRINTED IN THE UNITED STATES OF AMERICA

Author Disclaimer

This author disclaims any and all information provided in this book as it is not intended to treat or provide diagnoses.

This author, publisher, and any contributors, will not be liable for any potential damages as a result of following the information in this book.

There are potential risks associated with any nutritional and weight loss programs. While this author is a Registered Nurse, there has been no formal training in Nutrition or Exercise Science.

This author is fully aware that there is no knowledge of your particular and unique healthcare history.

Any lifestyle changes should always be discussed with a qualified healthcare provider.

This book is intended as a motivational tool. Consider your personal health history prior to changing your lifestyle.

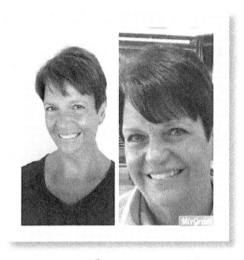

The photo on the left was
taken in September 2018.
125 pound weight reduction.

Dedication

This book is dedicated to my husband Marcel, our son Mike, grandsons Lucas and Ryan, and to my parents, Vinny and Sis Barricelli, in heaven. Their support and love have motivated me on this incredible journey toward a healthful life.

This book is also dedicated to Gin Stephens, intermittent fasting expert and author of Delay, Don't Deny and Feast Without Fear. Her guidance has been immeasurable.

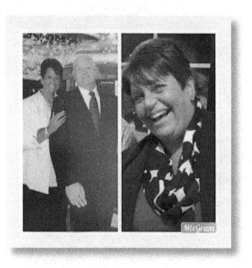

Left photo after 11 months
of intermittent fasting.
Down 100 pounds.

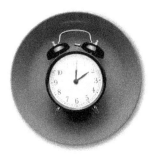

Acknowledgments

This book is motivational. It is not intended to provide medical advice. Please consult with a medical provider before implementing any weight loss program, fasting program, change in eating processes, or exercise plan.

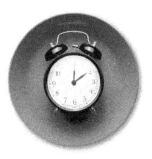

Introduction

This is a book about intermittent fasting. It is intended to be motivational and is not a health plan. I am not a physician. I am, however, a Registered Nurse with over 35 years of experience treating patients who have been impacted by weight-related problems. Before you embark on this quest, consult with a qualified medical provider who is familiar with your personal history.

You deserve a healthier lifestyle. You can change the way you eat and end the diet rollercoaster rides. If I could succeed with intermittent fasting, you can too.

I have dropped over 100 pounds in the last eighteen months by intermittent fasting and have never felt better. I share my story in the hope that it inspires you to change your life in the way I changed mine.

My intention is not to provide you with meal plans, recipes, or lists of calories. Haven't we had enough of that? You purchased this book for a reason. My hunch is you are tired of being overweight. Be prepared to unlearn what you have been taught about dieting and nutrition. This book will help guide you to begin the best journey of your life toward better health.

Like many, I thought the low-calorie, low-fat, low-cholesterol, dietary dogma was absolute truth. It was a blatant lie that was never based on factual data. The nutrition and diet worlds are engorged with money behind the smoke and mirrors.

For forty years, I tried numerous weight loss programs which I will describe. I started my first diet as a teenager. I restricted fats and calories most of my adult life. I faithfully exercised. I did yo-yo dieting from my teens until my fifties. I always lost weight like a rock star, and then gained pounds with a counterblow. Sound familiar?

We do not lack willpower or fortitude. We are strong and we are certainly not lazy. Heck no! For the first time in our painstakingly dieted lives, you will learn that intermittent fasting affords hope. Welcome to the blame free club toward a healthier you. We are so worth it! Consider us to be cleared of all "charges" related to being overweight. We have found a real solution. This is our "get out of jail free card."

This is a new-day for those who need to lose pounds and get healthier. Intermittent fasting is our sunrise. With intermittent fasting, our bodies are able to burn own body fat for energy. Fast, burn your body fat, lose weight, get healthier. Whether you want to lose 5, 10, 25, 50, 100, or more than 100 pounds, this book can guide you. The paradigm related to weight loss has shifted. Weight loss science is evolving to where it makes sense. Conventional diet mentality has been severely flawed for decades. Thank goodness we are catching on. May the intermittent fast be with all of you.

I will share resources who are champions among the intermittent fasting community. Gin Stephens, author of the book, *Delay, Don't Deny*, forever changed my life and the lives of thousands. I am eternally grateful to her for delivering the intermittent fasting message in a way that made it seem achievable.

I will describe intermittent fasting, insulin resistance, and low-carbohydrate high-fat diets. You will learn that dietary fat is longer forbidden in the food chain. This is not a typographical error. Butter is welcomed back with open arms....and it is incredibly decadent and delicious.

In the 1950's, it was believed that heart disease was spiraling to epidemic proportions. The hypothesis was that fat and cholesterol were to blame for the uptick in cardiac deaths. Physicians touted diets low in fat, low in cholesterol, and low in calories. These diets caught on and the nation bought the pitch with little supporting evidence. We believed it hook, line, and sinker. We heard low-fat and low-cholesterol from the government, the food industry, the pharmaceutical giants, and the media outlets. We were confident that they were all correct.

Yet, people grew fatter and unhealthier. Fats in our diets were akin to the Grinch Who Stole Christmas. Our waistlines enlarged, and low-fat foods became our coveted food superheroes. Snack cakes, deli flats masquerading as bread, low-fat cheeses, fat-free milk that resembled white water, margarine sprays pretending to be butter.....you get the vivid picture.

We were instructed to eat six times a day to "boost our metabolisms." How did that work for you? What was left to eat when we were told that fats and cholesterol were unacceptable? Sugars and processed foods of course. That's right, we were told to hold the avocado, but to load up on "heart healthy" grains, as one example. The packet of powdered oatmeal that I am holding is partially genetically modified and contains more sugar (32 grams) than a jelly-filled donut (18 grams). I'm going with the avocado and its whole and unprocessed healthy fats.

The American Heart Association (AHA) advised us to consume pasta, bread, grains, cereal, and starchy vegetables. We were told to restrict red meats, eggs, butter, whole milk, and creams. Our diets were overflowing with carbohydrates, and low-fat, low-calorie, low-taste, "knockoff" foods.

We counted calories, portions, and we wanted it if it was labeled as fat-free, low-fat, or healthy. We ate margarine instead of butter because it was marketed as healthier. Must be good right?

Ditch the hydrogenated oils and keep the trans fats low. Bring back the butter.

We were confident that avoiding egg yolks, butter, bacon, and eating breakfasts of cereal, fruit, and fat-free milk were going to help us lose weight like "champions." Breakfast is the most important meal of the day isn't it? If we don't eat, we will slow our metabolisms. Isn't that what we have heard? It is simply false and we now know better.

Have you ever seen the "heart healthy" labeling on various processed foods? Walk in the breakfast aisle at any grocery store. Pick up a plain packaged bagel? Most "heart healthy" breakfast foods (cereal, oatmeal, granola, bagels), contain more sugar than that donut. Sugar explosions made with processed flour, sugar, and genetically modified oils. I prefer eggs with butter and bacon instead please. Oh, and add some full-fat cheddar.

Be honest...How many Mondays have your started your diet in earnest? Come on, be honest. How many times have you felt there was something wrong with you because you give it all you've got but can't stick to it? How many times have you started the mighty diet, and then hit a dreaded plateau? Have you ever stopped trying to lose weight because you're tired of failing? I know I did. How many times have you been told by a medical provider to eat less and exercise more? Have you ever seen a medical provider for a minor ailment, only to be reminded you need to lose weight? Thank you, we know we are overweight but we are here because we sprained our wrist. Why can we develop self-driving cars, but not determine how to get the obesity curve to decline?

Have you ever replaced your big clothes (I get it...we have clothes in a variety of sizes) because they were too tight? Did they shrink in the closet because of the humidity? Sound familiar?

Anyone who needs to lose weight can relate. These are commonplace experiences. They certainly were for me. It is time to change. Intermittent fasting is transformative. This book has been written to guide you to become a timekeeper along your own weight loss journey.

The following experts have worked tirelessly to help us to change our approach to achieving weight loss and better health. Their books have become my inspiration, as well as inspiration to thousands. They have provided me with the necessary tools to write this book. I highly suggest the works from these amazing authors:

- *AC: The Power of Appetite Correction*, Bert Herring, MD, 2015.
- *Delay, Don't Deny*, Gin Stephens, 2016.
- *Feast Without Fear*, Gin Stephens, 2017.
- *Good Calories, Bad Calories*, Gary Taube, 2007.
- *Keto Clarity*, Jimmy Moore with Eric Westman, MD, 2014.
- *The Complete Guide to Fasting,* Jason Fung, MD, and Jimmy Moore, 2016.
- *The Fast-5 Diet*, Bert Herring, MD, 2005.
- *The Obesity Code: Unlocking the Secrets of Weight Loss*, Jason Fung, MD, 2016.
- *The Science of Skinny*, Dee McCaffrey, 2012.
- *The Big Fat Surprise*, Nina Teicholz, 2014.

Important Acronyms

The intermittent fasting community has a distinct language. Refer to this list for common acronyms you will see as you dive into the literature.

ACV	Apple Cider Vinegar
ADF	Alternate Day Fasting
BMI	Body Mass Index
BMR	Basal Metabolic Rate
BPC	Bullet Proof Coffee
CICO	Calories In/Calories Out
EF	Extended Fast
GHEE	Clarified Butter
HWC	Heavy Whipping Cream
IF	Intermittent Fasting
IR	Insulin Resistance
KETO	Ketogenic Diet
LCHF	Low Carb/High Fat
MACROS	Macronutrients
NSV	Non Scale Victory
SAD	Standard American Diet
WINDOW	Hours of Eating
WOE	Way of Eating
WOL	Way of Living
16:8, 18:8, 19:5, 20:4, 21:3, 22:2, 23:1	The first number is the fasted hours. The second number is the eating hours "window."

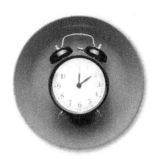

Table of Contents

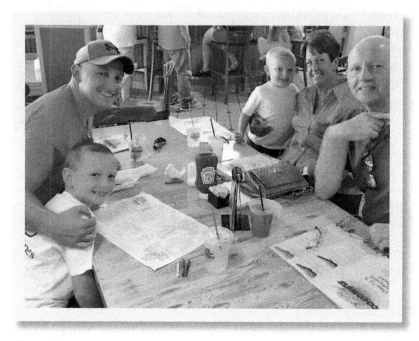

From left to right:
Lucas, Mike, Ryan, me, Marcel

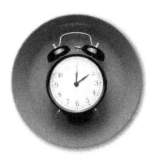

Chapter One
My Weight Loss Story

I am a 61 year old wife, mother, and Nana to two beautiful boys, Lucas (age 8), and Ryan (age 4). Health as the matriarch of this family is my motivation. Aren't we all worthy of better health?

This book is a claim to victory from being fat and unfit. Ditch your diet mentality today. Conventional diets are detrimental to long-term weight loss. It is a simple fact. Being fat is not about your willpower. There is hope.

My issues with weight started decades ago. I am 5'10" tall and was always large. Going through high school in the 1970's, there were limited diet plans available. Mainly, those who wanted to shed pounds, ate celery, grapefruit, and salad. My doctor prescribed caffeine-based diet pills and for the first time in my life, I became thin. I lost 50 pounds in a matter of months. I lived on low-fat cereal, "skim" milk, fish sticks because they were low-calorie and I could eat four as a portion, and elbow pasta because it made "a lot" when cooked. Pathetic right? Food was seldom enjoyable and I always felt deprived. Counting what you eat is tedious work.

I felt horrible on those diet pills but I was thin. Heart palpitations resulted and my diet pill phase ended abruptly. And back came the

50 pounds with a vengeance. At age 18, I was a diet failure. Luckily I was tall so was able to hide my bulges better than others.

College years brought more challenges. As a nursing student who lived on campus, my diet consisted of Ramen Noodles, burgers, fries, pizza, takeout Chinese, and of course wine. To feel healthy, I ate from the cafeteria salad bar. I piled my plates with croutons, potato salad, coleslaw, cheese, salami, and thick sugary dressings labeled as low-fat. It was salad with low-fat dressing after all. Wasn't that good for me?

I graduated from college in 1979 as a Registered Nurse. My husband, Marcel and I married shortly after graduation. Life was fantastic. I have the most supportive and loving partner on the planet. He loves me for who I am, despite my clothing size. Our early years consisted of entertaining, dining out with family and friends, and trying new dishes at home. We were living a beautiful life.

My wedding gown was a size 16 and I was close to ordering my dress from the plus-size rack. I starved myself before the fittings by cutting down my fish stick portions. My gosh! I truly sound crazy. Imagine being the bride and needing to get your gown from the fat-sized rack with three dresses to choose from? There was no online shopping in 1979.

I began my career as a RN working the evening shift in a large hospital. I loved the job and my work team. The hours, however, were tough. My diet morphed into fast food burgers at midnight while charting, takeout pizza, and microwavable leftovers. The fried veggie bar at work was a treat because after all, it was just vegetables. And my weight skyrocketed. Our son, Mike, was born in 1986 and we were blessed beyond words with a #perfectlife.

My goal was to shed the weight quickly, but life got difficult. My beloved mother, Sis, was battling end-stage cancer. Her cancer had spread to her bones and to her spinal cord. She was wheelchair bound and my father, Vinny, Marcel, and I provided home care for her. Working a full-time job, being a mother of a small child, and providing care for my mother, were stressful moments in our lives. Food brought comfort. My mother's passing in 1988 changed our entire world. My dear mother and friend was gone, and food was something we shared. And with comfort food, came pounds for me.

Being brought up in an Italian household, food was a vehicle to demonstrate love. We always enjoyed large Sunday dinners at Vinny's to share our weeks, and to celebrate our love with tasty concoctions. Vinny was an incredible cook and he never skimped on ingredients. We ate eggplant parmesan, steaks, ribs, chicken, shrimp, always pasta, and desserts made of milk chocolate and whipped cream. We never went without quality food and we celebrated the bonds we had as a loving family. One of the staples on our table was fresh Italian bread. Vinny bought that bread from the finest bakeries and it was always the star of the show. And my weight climbed. It was time for a plan to get healthier. This lifelong dieter needed to regain control.

I tried a popular "counting diet" many times. I will not diet-bash in this book and my comments are written generically. I always lost significant weight, but never liked the program and to be honest, I wondered if it worked long-term, why did I need to restart on so many Mondays? I thought food was supposed to be enjoyed? Every time I stopped "watching," the weight came back. Little did I know I had dropped my Basal Metabolic Rate (BMR) with each attempt. Even eating "healthy," I was destined to gain. I wish I knew back then that it was not my fault.

Now that I have changed my own life and dropped over 100 pounds, I realize that counting food does not incentivize us to keep weight off permanently. How could diet plans make money if it was a once and done process? And while I love famous diet spokespersons, let's be honest guys. Many have not conquered their own weight battles despite personal trainers and in-house chefs. Enough

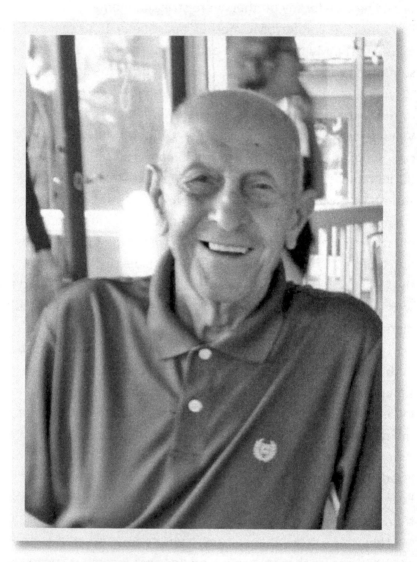

My amazing father,
Vincent Barricelli at age 93.

said, you get it!

During the next few decades, I played the diet game like a ping-pong match. I tossed the same 50 pounds back and forth like Lucas and Ryan's soccer ball. I then discovered a diet plan with prepackaged foods and face-to-face coaching. I paid hundreds of dollars to lose 50 pounds, and to be guided by "counselors." I succeeded! I lost that weight in three months, eating prepackaged, tasteless, chemically-laden "Frankenfoods." Truly the most repugnant things I have ever had the displeasure of eating. After nine months of cardboard rounds resembling "pizza," diet gelatin, and thousands of dollars ultimately spent, I quit. Prepackaged foods were getting old. Our son, Mike, was a talented soccer and baseball player, and life was filled with family, friends, and social gatherings. My plan was to keep the weight off by counting calories again. Or so I thought.

Any surprise that the pounds packed on once I started eating real food? Heck no, I was determined not to go backwards. I was brimming with willpower and determination. Marcel supported the prepackaged food plan and the thousands of dollars I had spent would NOT be in vain. I am a very driven person and when I get something in my head, I make it happen.

I had a "brilliant" idea (or so I thought at the time). I started protein shakes, and a diet that consisted of popcorn rice cakes, fake bread rounds, veggie soy burgers, frozen soy "chicken," fat-free, low-calorie, and tasteless foods. If it was fat-free, I ate it. If it was low-calorie, I counted it. I could not lose additional weight no matter how much willpower I had. So, I did what many dieters do. I cut back even more on calories. If I topped 1000 calories daily, that was a lot. Did I lose? I lost very little and I was desperate. I was determined. What was wrong with me? I was maxed out on dieting.

I was tired of avoiding family photos. I was worn out from feeling sluggish. I was exhausted from avoiding social gatherings because they were stressful. I was a true #dietfailure. So, I added vigorous exercise to my plan. How could I be consuming less than 1000 calories daily and not losing weight? I certainly had determination and strength. I was not going to quit. Exercise, I thought, was the only answer. We bought our first treadmill. I was so out of shape that Marcel stood with me while I accomplished 2 laps or 0.5 miles. That's right, doing ½ a mile was strenuous for my overly dieted body. But, I kept at it with the utmost determination to win the battle. I succeeded. I began losing weight again. And with each 10 pounds I dropped, Marcel reminded me that I had lost a ten pound sack of potatoes. It felt great and exercise became our passion. Today, we have an in-house gym with his and her treadmills (how sweet), a weight bench, free weights, and a yoga section. How life has changed...from cupcakes and corn chips to daily yoga and ninety minute workouts. Marcel's guidance and continuous support pulled me through. Have I mentioned how wonderful he is?

When I said exercise was "vigorous," I meant vigorous. I did a combination of cardio and weight training three times daily. That is right, daily. I lived on low-calorie, low-fat foods with three times daily exercise for 10 years. I lost over 100 pounds. But it got hard to keep it going. I played the diet game and always tossed 50 pounds out of the 100 pounds back and forth. Then life, as we know it can, got in the way.

In 2012, I became diet and exercise drained. No matter how little I ate, or how much I worked out, I gained. In order to even maintain my weight loss, my body was expecting three times daily workouts and less than 1000 calories of food. Little did I know I had lowered my Basal Metabolic Rate (BMR) drastically. I was overly dieted and overly exercised.

Basal Metabolic Rate (BMR) is the rate at which our bodies use energy at rest for functions like breathing and keeping warm. My dieting caused my BMR to tank. The harder I tried, the worse I did.

I fell into the mindset that if I worked out, I could eat more. I got up every morning at 4 a.m. to exercise before work. Instead of lunch at the hospital, I went for a walk. If I had a meeting, I walked to the location. After work, Marcel and I went for another walk. He supported me each day. We walked in rain, wind, snow, 95 degrees, and 10 degrees. We wore reflector vests in winter, and carried bug repellent in summer. Walking was life and the only things that stopped us were ice storms and lightning. Yes, we walked in rain and snow. The reality, however, is that exercise is beneficial, but it will not negate bad eating habits. And my inner food beast reared her ugly head because I thought I had earned it. Exercise does not change the fact that you can dig your grave with your own fork. We cannot outrun the plate even if we think we can.

In March of 2014, life took an unexpected and nearly fatal turn.

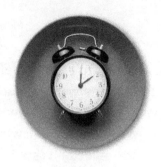

Chapter Two
Life Changing Illness

On March 21, 2014, life would be forever changed. I am fortunate that I am alive to tell the story. Marcel and I had returned from a Caribbean cruise. We were happy, rested, tanned, and of course, fatter. Marcel is blessed with being able to eat whatever he wishes and still wears the same size he did when we married, 39 years ago.

Shortly after our return, I developed Norovirus. Norovirus is a contagious virus that causes nausea, vomiting, and diarrhea. What a way to get rid of the cruise pounds! For a week, I could not eat, drink, or workout. Italian Ice was my salvation. Then out of nowhere, I developed leg pains.

Having been so sick, I assumed the pain was viral. Within a few days, I became short of breath with even simple activities. I could not walk on a flat surface without gasping for breath. But life is unpredictable. My aunt Rose passed away. Rose was my father's sister and an important member of our family. I needed to be strong to support my family. I went to the funeral with my shortness of breath, and figured it was all related to the virus. I told myself to push through and tough it out. Not exactly a smart plan, especially for a nurse. When the funeral concluded and I knew that my father was ok, I went to the Emergency Department, struggling to catch my breath. I assumed I had a respiratory virus and would be discharged with an inhaler and a steroid.

The Emergency Department confirmed the unthinkable. I had developed extensive "saddle" pulmonary emboli (blood clots) in both lungs. They believed that dehydration caused by the virus, coupled with sudden immobility, and the recent flight home from the cruise, were contributing factors. My resting pulse oximetry reading (measure of peripheral oxygen) was 70, which is life-threateningly low. I was almost placed on a ventilator. Bottom line was I almost did not survive. I spent four days in the ICU, underwent countless diagnostic tests, and was told that due to my vigorous exercise routine, my cardiovascular system was incredibly strong. They told me that one third of people with extensive clots like this do not survive to tell their story. I was told I was "the sickest patient in the ICU." Yikes, I'm pretty sure nobody ever wants to hear those words in a large hospital with many ICU patients who looked much sicker than me. I was in my fifties and had just returned from the Caribbean.

What? They must have read the CT Scan incorrectly. The pulse oximeter must have been malfunctioning. I had just gotten off a ship and was tanned and healthy. They were spot on with the diagnosis and I was blessed with a second chance at life. I survived and was able to learn from the experience.

I was evaluated by heart and lung specialists. The pulmonologist discharged me on a blood thinner. I was told that being overweight was a risk factor in developing more blood clots. Here we go again. Another thing that being overweight contributes to. The side effects of obesity never seem to end.

While I was in the ICU, my family was the basis of my recovery. My husband's smile guided me through this storm. His strength and love were the comfort that pulled me through. In the tough times, we grow stronger as a family. Our adult son, Mike, is kind, nurturing, caring, and truly an incredible person. One of the greatest comforts was to see first-hand the person our son had become in this time of need.

Our now 4 year old grandson, Ryan, was not born at the time. The reality was that I almost did not get to meet him. That rocked me to my very core. My motivation to get healthier was for my own life, and also for them. My grandson, Lucas, (age 4 at the time) picked up my photo and cried. He "did not want Nana to be in the hospital." And home was where I was going to be. Coloring eggs and making decorations with my little buddy Lucas.

Seeing sweet Lucas holding my picture was my forever moment. The moment where motivation to live healthier was strong as iron. If there was a way to get healthier, I was determined to follow it. This became my long-term goal throughout the intermittent fasting process.

There was no question. I would survive the blood clots, and I would do everything in my power to reduce the chances that they would return. Since being overweight increased the risk of clots, it was time to change. Weight loss failure was done and I was going to find success.

My plan was to start another calorie-restricted diet on Monday.

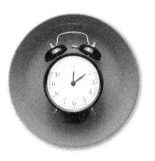

Chapter Three
It's An App

*H*aving survived the blood clots, it was time to make serious changes. I did research and discovered a free calorie-tracking application. I downloaded the application (app) and committed to the plan. It was simple to use, tracked foods, exercise, weights, calories, and the menu of food choices was extensive. The app recommended a "calorie budget" based on your weight and your weight loss goals. It seemed too good to be true. Of course I could do this. And I did.

When the holidays rolled around, my food beast returned. The indulgences returned. Once again, it was hard to get back into the calorie-counting drudgery. My mindset was on celebrating, not on restricting.

And then, my Dad, Vinny, passed away in January of 2016. Vinny was the light of our lives. He was thoughtful, charming, loved by everyone that knew him, and to many, he was the "unofficial mayor" of our town. His passing hit our family like a ton of bricks. It was difficult to pick another Monday start-date during this period of grief.

Like many of us, regardless of the diet we choose, we start with the best intentions. We have willpower and determination. We pick our Monday with dread, eat like dragons on Sunday, and ultimately lose weight. At about the six to twelve month point, we get fed up with deprivation, and the tasteless low-calorie foods we eat to drop those pounds. We feel hungry and we do not enjoy meals. So... we "cheat." We get tired of the flat deli rounds that we call "rolls." We think we were destined to be overweight, that it is our fault, and once again, we quit. Gosh, this is hard. Sound familiar?

My food beast controlled me until the Summer of 2016. I got back into the tracking app. This time, however, I did something I have never done before. I joined the online Facebook support-group. My life would be forever changed by the fellowship I became part of. I loved being able to work on this goal with other people who were like me.

I followed the app, connected with thousands of people, and felt a connection. We discussed victories, challenges, temptations, tips, and stumbling blocks. I transitioned from a person needing support, to someone who enjoyed providing inspiration to others. The online support group was a safe haven for the next six months. The support group, and my calorie-restricted diet, felt good and comfortable. I lost some weight but when we went on our annual cruise in 2017, the application, like every other diet plan, felt way too restrictive, and I stopped again.

The lightning bolt moment at the end of that vacation, changed my life. While I usually hid from pictures, in this one, I was front, center, and more than visible. Pictures do not lie.

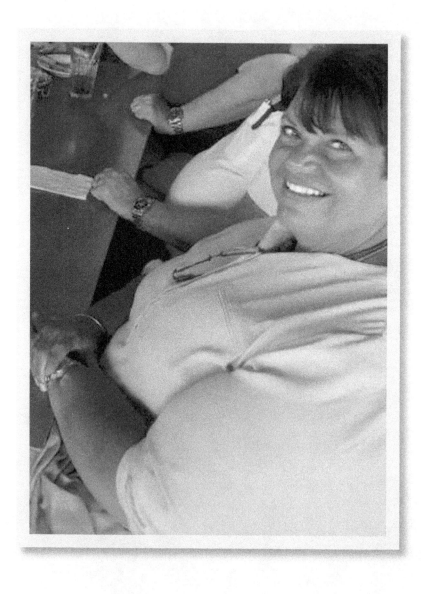

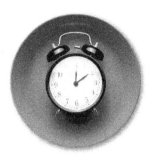

Chapter Four
Lightning Bolt Moment

Something happened to encourage you to start your weight loss journey. You were motivated to buy this book. Was it a photo? Is it an upcoming vacation or special event? Do you feel unwell? Did your weight reach a new high? Are your big clothes feeling tight?

Something sparked you to search for inspiration. Something inside of you may have been your lightning bolt moment. Your moment can change your life. Mine did. Let me remind you that we are not destined for failure.

My lightning bolt moment was this photo. I know, it sounds cliché. Marcel and I were at a restaurant with friends. The waiter snapped a photo of our group and the photo was posted. Oh my goodness! My arm looked like a watermelon. My neck was the size of a soccer ball. My cheeks looked like a pie. How did this happen? Was that really me? Was the camera distorted? I was not able to stand in the back of this photo. There were no plants nearby to hide behind. Darn it!

I needed to make changes quickly. This change had to be a lifestyle change, not another calorie-counting conundrum. How many more times could I try and ultimately fail to get this weight off? Oh by the way, in the photo, we were eating fried cheese. Of course we were.

As fate would have it, I saw a promotion regarding Dr. Jason Fung's book, *"The Obesity Code."* I also received a prompt for a book by an intermittent fasting expert, Gin Stephens, *"Delay, Don't Deny."* I bought both books in 2017, and started extensive research on intermittent fasting (IF). The more I read, the more it made sense in my skeptical brain. I was sparked with optimism. Being a nurse, I am accustomed to exploring research. The future seemed promising. As I studied the science behind intermittent fasting, I knew this was the answer-the missing link to my weight problems. Thank you Dr. Fung and Gin Stephens for saving my life. I did not know at the time that Gin Stephens would be the primary person behind my personal success. She has guided me through her mentorship, expert knowledge of intermittent fasting, and her friendship.

Many doctors tell us to lose weight by eating less and moving more. Sounds simple doesn't it? According to the Centers for Disease Control and Prevention (CDC), "The prevalence of obesity is 39.8% and affects about 93.3 million of US adults." https://www.cdc.gov/obesity/data/adult.html.

People lose weight on popular diet programs, yet 93.3 million US adults are still obese. Staggering numbers!

According to, https://fatfu.wordpress.com/2008/01/24/weight-watchers , "two out of a thousand...who reach goal weight (by counting diets) stayed there for more than five years." I don't know about you but even with exercise three times daily, I was never one of the chosen two out of the thousand. Were you?

Losing weight is not about counting calories for the long haul. Fat is not the enemy in the food chain. All calories are not created equally. The body is fueled much better by a 150 calorie sweet potato than a one ounce serving of "Flamin Hot Cheetos" at 160 calories. Our meals do not have to be tasteless and lean. Losing weight should not be about fitting into an outfit, or looking svelte for vacation. We do not have to load up our plates with food guilt.

Losing weight needs to be a lifestyle health improvement plan. Bingo! That is the basis for success. This needs to be a lifelong plan. Get ready to start refining your timekeeper skills because you are going to need them.

As I stated earlier, dieting has been part of my life since my teens. My guess is that many of you relate. People lose weight on diets over the first six to twelve months. They love their programs when they lose. They believe they are on the "best diet" in the world because they are losing weight and celebrities endorse them. They blame themselves, however, when they gain it back.

- 🕐 Why aren't we told that calorie-restricted diets lower our metabolisms and that we may regain that weight?
- 🕐 Why don't they tell us that even if we restrict calories forever, we will still gain weight? Sorry folks, it is a proven fact. It is a sound business model for most weight loss plans.
- 🕐 Our obesity equals their soaring profit margins!
- 🕐 Have you ever gone off your diet on a vacation? Is it easy to get back into the groove? Of course not. It's super hard!
- 🕐 Restrictions lead to binging because life happens, and we are humans. Once we binge, it is very difficult to tame that food beast within us. My beast used to scream for Twinkies by the way.
- 🕐 Counting food is tolerable at first. Eventually it becomes tedious. Without fixing that root cause of our weight problem, counting will fail long-term.
- 🕐 Calories in/calories out (CI/CO) plans are effective for short-term success, but behavior toward food does not improve by deprivation.

Did you know that most food I ate on CI/CO diets was low-fat, processed, 100 calorie snack bags, and microwavable meals packed with chemicals and preservatives? I thought weird manufactured bars labeled as "healthy" were treats. Not exactly a wholesome way to live. My diet cycle was, lose weight, feel incredibly proud, go off the diet, have trouble getting back, and regain my weight with a few more "bonus" pounds. My hunch is that many of you feel these words to the tips of your toes. And when we fail, the diet industry gets richer.

My prepackaged food diet was convenient. There are several of these plans out there and I will not criticize a particular plan. I was told what to eat, and how much to eat. Portions in foil vacuum packs were miniscule. Yes, I lost weight at first. The problem was that life is not about prepackaged, chemically-laden, tiny rations called "food." The foods, to me, were tasteless, bland, and lacked quality nutrition. While I lost weight as many people do, the plan was not sustainable despite their spokespersons' claims to thinner bodies. And, it became pricey! "Hey family, want to come over for dinner?" Wait, let me heat up my pathetic and tasteless pizza round. Ugh! You get the picture.

Meal replacement shakes were my next brilliant idea. Yes, I lost pounds once again. Bravo! Living life swallowing chalk-like shakes was revolting. Is that the way you want to live your healthy life forever? I thought food was supposed to be enjoyed.

Food should be enjoyable and as close to its natural state as possible. Foods are better for our health when they are not overly processed and modified. Run from prepackaged food plans Forest... RUN! I loved Forest Gump by the way....

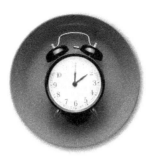

Chapter Five
Count Hours Not Calories

A ccording to the Weight Management Center at Boston Medical Center, (https://bmc.org/nutrition-and-weight-management/weight-management), "An estimated 45 million Americans go on a diet each year, and spend $33 billion each year on weight loss products." Despite this, two-thirds of Americans are obese or overweight. I certainly was! I am tired of playing the game and padding their bottom lines, along with padding my own waistline. Are you tired of it as well?

Let's try counting only the time we eat. Let's restrict the hours we eat by intermittent fasting. Let's become fat burners. Let's stop counting calories and depriving ourselves of food we love. Let's enjoy meals again.

Intermittent fasting is the missing link in our dieted lives. It makes sense! No matter how dedicated we have been to calories in/calories out (CI/CO) diets, how hard we have tried, or how faithfully we have exercised, we lose pounds and inevitably gain them back. We feel amazing when we lose and see progress. In about a year, most of us are back where we started. If you're like me, you may even have added more pesky pounds and it gets tiring.

Intermittent fasting will change your life. Intermittent fasting has allowed me to shed over 100 pounds in the past eighteen months. Don't worry-fasting is not a fad. It has been followed for religious and cultural traditions throughout the world for centuries.

Reminder Checklist

- ◷ We are not lazy overeaters with zero willpower.
- ◷ We are not at fault for being overweight.
- ◷ We are strong.
- ◷ We are hopeful that our weight battles can be conquered.
- ◷ We should try intermittent fasting and it is free of charge. Please consult with a qualified medical provider who knows your medical history first.
- ◷ We are ready to get healthier and lose weight!
- ◷ Ready, set, go.......
- ◷ Start counting the hours when you eat and stop counting calories.
- ◷ Repeat after me, food freedom and fat burning rule!
- ◷ You are so worth it!

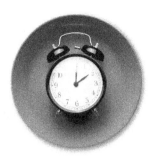

Chapter Six

What Is Intermittent Fasting (IF)?

1. IF reaches beyond conventional diets and changes the times we eat.
2. IF is a health plan that allows us to enjoy real food, lose weight, and get healthier.
3. IF makes healthy eating tasty and delicious again.
4. IF simplifies life and it is free of charge. There are fewer meals to buy and prepare.
5. IF cycles between eating "windows" and fasting times.
6. IF has been practiced by spiritual groups and by our ancestors throughout history.

Types of Intermittent Fasting

a. **Time Restricted Eating** involves choosing a fasting period and an eating "window." This is the most popular type of IF. An eating window is when you are able to eat.
b. **Different Time Restricted Eating Combinations:**
   16:8 is 16 fasted hours with an 8 hour window.
   17:7 is 17 fasted hours with a 7 hour window.
   18:6 is 18 fasted hours with a 6 hour window.

19:5 is 19 fasted hours with a 5 hour window.

20:4 is 20 fasted hours with a 4 hour window.

21:3 is 21 fasted hours with a 3 hour window.

22:2 is 22 fasted hours with a 2 hour window.

23:1 is 23 fasted hours with a 1 hour window.

c. **5:2 Method** involves fasting two nonconsecutive days each week. On fast days, you can eat 500 to 600 calories. The other 5 days you eat normally. While many people find success with 5:2, I found the fasted days were very difficult.

d. **Extended Fasting (EF)** involves no food intake, other than water, black coffee, or tea, for an extended time-frame. I will not discuss EF in this book but words of caution-any fasts greater than 72 hours should always be medically supervised for your safety.

e. **Alternate Day Fasting (ADF)** involves eating one day and fasting the next. Many eat 500 to 600 calories on fast days. I was not successful with ADF, as I tended to over-eat on my feeding days.

f. **One Meal A Day (OMAD)** involves eating one true meal daily. OMAD is a very common form of intermittent fasting. This is my chosen version of intermittent fasting.

7. IF improves cells within our bodies in the following ways:

a. Levels of the hormone insulin drop when we fast. Lower insulin allow us to use our body fat for fuel. We become fat burners instead of sugar burners. In intermittent fasting, fat burners WIN.

b. Human Growth Hormone (HGH) spikes which allows us to gain lean muscle mass. Refer to https://www.diet-doctor.com/fasting-and-growth-hormone.

c. Basal metabolic rates increase by 4-14% by the release of the hormone noradrenaline. This prevents the dreaded "starvation mode " that can occur in calorie-restricted diets. Read the difference between calorie restriction and fasting according to Intensive Dietary Management: in this fascinating post: https://idmprogram.com/difference-calorie-restriction-fasting-fasting-27/

    d. Fasted cells recycle cellular "garbage." This is called Autophagy (pronounced Aut-toph-a-gee). The 2016 Nobel Prize in Medicine was awarded for this discovery to Yoshinori Ohsumi.

    e. Hormones play big roles in weight control. Leptin controls when we feel satiated (full). Insulin is a fat storage hormone, as we have discussed. Glucagon stimulates the liver to release its stored glycogen, and ghrelin lets us know when we are hungry. Intermittent fasting "tunes-up" these hormones so that they can work more efficiently.

8. IF has added health benefits besides weight loss:
   a. IF enhances the ability to enjoy food you love.
   b. IF is flexible, convenient, and free of charge.
   c. IF works with the foods that make YOU feel good.
   d. IF increases mental focus and clarity.
   e. IF increases energy.
   f. IF increases ability to burn fat stores.
   g. IF can reduce triglycerides, blood sugar, LDL cholesterol and insulin resistance.
   h. IF reduces risk of prediabetes and type 2 diabetes.
   i. IF can prevent some cancers.
   j. IF increases certain brain hormones and can protect against Alzheimer's Disease.
   k. IF reverses the aging process.

9. IF is NOT for everyone.
   a. IF is **not for you** if you have a history of an eating disorder.

b. IF is not for you if you are very underweight.
c. IF is not recommended for women who are pregnant or breastfeeding, or who are trying to conceive.
d. IF is not suggested in certain hormonal disorders or adrenal fatigue.
e. As with any new weight loss, diet, or fitness program, it is advisable to discuss IF with a qualified healthcare provider who is aware of your personal medical history.
f. People who have low blood pressure, type 1 or type 2 diabetes, gout, trouble controlling their blood sugars, or who take prescribed medications for various medical conditions, must discuss IF with a qualified healthcare provider before starting.
g. Children 18 years of age and younger should not practice IF.

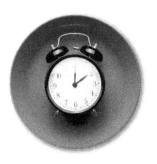

Chapter Seven
OMAD

*Y*ou cannot read about intermittent fasting without seeing the abbreviation OMAD. OMAD is the acronym for One Meal A Day. OMAD means you limit eating to a specified timeframe and eat one true meal. Despite what the food marketers have told us, we have never been designed to eat all day. We are used to eating frequently throughout the day because that is what we have been advised to do. Our bodies are conditioned to expect that food. Have you ever eaten a bagel and fruit for breakfast and by noon, you are ready to chew your arm off if you don't get that burger?

OMAD is defined as having one true meal daily.

1. OMAD can be a safe and effective way to lose weight.
2. OMAD is free and saves time.
3. OMAD could be a five or six hour window with one snack, one meal, and one dessert.
4. OMAD is flexible.
5. OMAD means you eat and plan one true meal a day.
6. OMAD allows you to eat your main meal when it suits your lifestyle.

7. OMAD does not need to be eaten within one hour.
8. OMAD is my chosen intermittent fasting plan. For me, I enjoy one true meal, a light snack, and sometimes a dessert.

OMAD tips: Eat your OMAD when you are hungry and within your eating window. Ensure that your plate is balanced with nutrient-rich food. Add healthy fats to your meal (butter, olive oil, cheese, sour cream, etc.), to keep you satiated. Consume vegetables, proteins, carbs, and enough fiber to achieve satiety. Your one meal can be a feast.

Please do not gorge yourself. OMAD is easy to adhere to but it is not a free-pass to stuff ourselves. While an occasional drive-through meal is fine, diets loaded with highly processed foods can contribute to heart disease, elevated cholesterol, depression, high blood pressure, insulin resistance, bloating, blood sugar elevations, etc.

Read more at https://www.healthline.com/health/fast-food-effects-on-body.

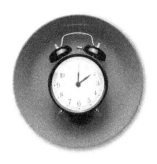

Chapter Eight
Insulin Resistance

According to www.endocrineweb.com, one in three Americans, including half of those age 60 and older, are insulin resistant, (https://www.endocrineweb.com/conditions/type-2-diabetes/insulin-resistance-causes-symptoms.)

More than 84 million American adults are prediabetic, according to the National Institute of Health (NIH). 30 to 50% of these prediabetics will develop type 2 diabetes in their lifetimes.

Insulin is a hormone produced by a gland near the stomach called the pancreas. Normally, our bodies breakdown food and convert it into glucose. Glucose is usually the main source of energy for our bodies when we eat a standard diet. Insulin helps cells use that glucose for energy. In insulin resistance (IR), cells ignore signals to grab the glucose to use as fuel. Glucose builds in the bloodstream, causing blood sugars to rise.

When we eat frequently throughout the day, in people with insulin resistance, the pancreas has to work overtime to make more insulin to handle the constant food. Eventually, the pancreas gets worn out. Blood sugar rises and IR ultimately can lead to prediabetes and type 2 diabetes.

Welcome to The International Regency (IR) Hotel

This analogy should make insulin resistance simple to understand.

1. The hormone insulin is considered the *"key card"* to access your room.
2. Insulin, the *"key card"* must fit into the cell, the *"door"* to your room.
3. With insulin resistance, the *"key card"* (insulin) does not open the *"door"* (cell). You're stuck in the hallway of the IR Hotel.
4. Glucose in the blood is not allowed into the *"door"* (cell) because the *"key card"* (insulin) is faulty. The *"key card"* (insulin) needs reprogramming.
5. Glucose collects in the *"hallway"* (bloodstream). It cannot gain entry to the *"door"* (cell).
6. The *"front desk"* (pancreas) makes another *"key card"* (more insulin). The hope is that the new *"key card"* will open the *"door"* (cell). Glucose in the *"hallway"* (bloodstream) continues to builds up with nowhere to go. That glucose then gets stored as body fat because the cell refuses to use it properly.
7. Excess glucose hanging out in the *"hallway"* (bloodstream) contributes to prediabetes, and type 2 diabetes by elevating blood sugar levels.
8. Instead of using glucose in the way it is intended, glucose builds up in the blood. In type 1 diabetes, the pancreas does **not** make enough insulin. In type 2 diabetes and prediabetes, the pancreas makes **too much** insulin yet the cells are resistant to it.

If you do **not have type 1 diabetes**, why do we treat insulin resistance, prediabetes, and type 2 diabetes, with diets of 3 daily meals and snacks? Doesn't that cause more insulin to be produced? Doesn't that glucose continue to build in the bloodstream? Doesn't insulin convert to more body fat because we have not fixed the real problem - resistance to insulin? Aren't we making ourselves fatter by eating all the time?

Insulin blocks fat burning. Without correcting the broken *"key card"* (insulin), the *"door"* (cell) will not accept glucose from the food we eat. So, we get fatter. How can this get fixed? By fasting and by stopping the constant production of insulin caused by eating throughout the day.

Thank you Dr. Jason Fung, for enlightening us with your master-piece, *"The Obesity Code."* I highly suggest this revolutionary and life changing book on curing obesity. Dr. Fung is a Toronto-based nephrologist with a special interest in type 2 diabetes, and intermittent fasting. He is the founder of the Intensive Dietary Management (IDM) program.

1. Who is more likely to develop insulin resistance (IR)?
   b. Overweight and obese individuals.
   c. People age 45 and older.
   d. Those with poor dietary patterns who eat lots of overly processed foods.
   e. People with limited physical activity and a large waist size.
   f. People with a family history of diabetes.
   g. People with polycystic ovarian syndrome (PCOS).
   h. People with obstructive sleep apnea and sleep disorders.
   i. People with high blood pressure, elevated blood glucose and triglyceride levels.
   j. Those with non-alcoholic fatty liver disease (NAFLD) which increases the risk for liver damage and heart disease.

    k. People with skin tags and discolored dark skin patches mainly on the neck, arms, or legs (acanthosis nigricans).

2. How is insulin resistance diagnosed?

    a. Blood glucose levels (fasting blood glucose or hemoglobin A1C levels) are tested.

    b. Blood tests for insulin resistance are seldom performed and are used for research purposes.

    c. One in three Americans, including half of those age 60 and older, have insulin resistance.

    d. Wow! Yet we still advise people to eat three meals a day and frequent snacks. Is it any wonder we are getting fatter?

3. How can I prevent or reverse insulin resistance?

    a. By losing weight and by reducing the time we eat. When we fast, insulin is not produced. The liver relies on its glycogen stores for fuel. When the glycogen stores are depleted, the body turns to fat for fuel.

    b. Turning to our body fat for fuel is what we want!

4. How long does it take for your body to adjust to being fat adapted?

    a. When we fast, our body converts its major fuel source to ketones which are produced from fat.

    b. You can become fat adapted by intermittent fasting.

    c. You do not need to follow a low-carbohydrate diet to become fat adapted.

    d. Fat adaptation means you are using ketones, directly from fat for energy.

    e. This process can take several weeks to achieve. It took me 3 to 4 weeks to get there. Be patient because fat burning life is amazing.

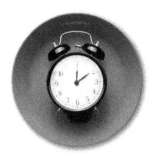

Chapter Nine
Manage Insulin Resistance

*L*et's toss conventional diet mentality to the curb. I have lost over 100 pounds and am proud to be fat adapted. I have conquered my resistance to insulin.

As stated, our bodies can be fueled in one of two ways.

1. We can burn glucose and be sugar burners.
2. We can burn fat and be fat burners.

Remember that being overweight is predominantly caused by the ineffectiveness of hormones, namely insulin. Intermittent fasting improves our resistance to insulin. Our weight has never been due to our lack of willpower. Ahh, that feels affirming to say that. Lose the fat shame right now and forever. You are forgiven!

What are the choices on the journey to drop weight and improve health?

1. Choice One
   We can restrict ourselves by eating low-fat, low-calorie foods, move more, eat throughout the day causing insulin to rise, further increase insulin resistance, increase blood

sugars, drop metabolic rates making it harder to keep weight off, and continue on this conventional dietary journey. Doesn't the mainstream advice we have received for fifty years tell us to do just this?

Has it worked long-term? If it worked, why are we getting fatter? Why are 93.3 million adults in the U.S. classified as obese. If this diet "wisdom" works, why is the obesity curve climbing like our waist sizes? I doubt your clothes shrunk in the closet on their own.

If Choice One worked, you would not have needed this book. By the way, thank you.

2. Choice Two
    We can open our minds to intermittent fasting. We can stop counting calories and start counting hours instead. We can limit when we eat and have freedom over food choices. We can lose more weight, will not drop basal metabolic rates, will lower insulin levels, will build lean body mass by increased HGH, will enhance energy and focus by increased noradrenaline, will be able to enjoy delicious meals that are not low-calorie or low-fat, will enjoy benefits of autophagy, will increase brain health, decrease inflammation, and will decrease the risk of certain cancers.

Does the better choice seem obvious? I would say an overwhelming YES to intermittent fasting.

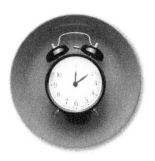

Chapter Ten
Low-Carbohydrate/High-Fat Diet

O besity is caused by the inability to regulate insulin. Obesity is not caused by a lack of determination. Regular CI/CO diets do not address the reason behind our weight issues. The billion dollar diet industry counts on this for profits.

When we eat, insulin spikes. The glucose that is not used by our cells is stored mainly in the liver as glycogen. The liver has limited storage. It's like my suitcase before a cruise...limited storage capacity.

When our glycogen storage is filled, the liver creates new fat because it cannot hold onto the excess. The liver runs out of space much like my suitcase runs out of space for another pair of sandals. Body fat, however, has a large storage tank. My thighs are proof that this is the true! For additional information, check out: https://medium.com/@drjasonfung/understanding-obesity -f233fbb38dc1.

When we fast, insulin drops.
- 🕐 Practice intermittent fasting.
- 🕐 Decrease insulin levels.

- 🕐 Breakdown glycogen in liver for energy.
- 🕐 When glycogen is depleted, fat is converted to energy in the form of ketone bodies.

When we eat, insulin levels rise.
- 🕐 Eat food.
- 🕐 Increase insulin levels. **Insulin blocks fat burning.**
- 🕐 Store glucose in liver as glycogen.
- 🕐 Fat is formed when liver glycogen storage "suitcase" gets filled.

When we do not correct the root cause of obesity (insulin), most people who lose weight will gain it back. Stop supporting the ever-growing weight loss industry if you want to lose the weight for good.

Did you ever experience a leaky basement? Vacuuming the water with a wet-vac fixes the problem temporarily. Until you repair the reason your basement leaked, you will always be vacuuming water following heavy rain. Vacuuming the basement repeatedly is like losing weight by counting calories. It is a short-term fix and guaranteed to fail for the long haul. Calorie counting does not address the root cause.

Low-carbohydrate, high-fat (LCHF) diets are often referenced in literature on intermittent fasting. There is a striking overlap between LCHF and intermittent fasting and there are similar features. They are weight loss first-cousins. There are various definitions for LCHF diets in the literature:

According to dietdoctor.com (https://www.dietdoctor.com/low-carb/keto/how-low-carb-is-keto), LCHF levels are grouped as follows:

1. Liberal LCHF = 50 to 100 carb grams daily.
2. Moderate LCHF = 20 to 50 carb grams daily.
3. Ketogenic LCHF = less than 20 carb grams daily. This is ultra-low carb.

Everyone who practices IF does not need to restrict carbohydrates (carbs) to burn fat. Intermittent fasting without carb restriction can reduce insulin and push the body to burn fat on its own. Restricting carbs, by eating a LCHF diet, may push the body to burn fat at a higher level for some people with severe insulin resistance.

Generally, a low-carb diet is defined as consuming less than 100 carb grams daily. According to Mayo Clinic, a standard diet of 2000 calories translates into 325 grams of carbs for those not restricting carbs. I'm pretty sure I consumed over that in Cheetos alone.

How do you know if you need to restrict carbs along with your intermittent fasting plan? How severely insulin resistant are you?

The longer you have been obese, the harder it may be to lose weight. While it is important to check with a qualified healthcare provider who is familiar with your history, intermittent fasting combined with LCHF can be a great choice for some of us:

1. People with type 2 diabetes.
2. People who have significant amounts of weight to lose (like me).
3. People who have been on numerous past diets where they restricted calories and ultimately lowered their metabolisms (like me).
4. People who have addictions to sugary sweets and refined carbs (grains that have been processed by a food manufacturer causing the fiber to no longer remain intact). Examples of refined carbs are white bread, sugar, white rice, pastry, white pasta, breakfast cereals, sugar-sweetened drinks, and more. The American Journal of Clinical Nutrition states that, "fast-digesting carbohydrates can stimulate regions of the brain involved in cravings and addiction," (https://www.npr.org/sections/thesalt/2013/06/26/195292850/can-you-be-addicted-to-carbs).

It is possible to achieve results from intermittent fasting without restricting carbs. For me, due to many past diets, I was strongly insulin resistant. I had over 100 pounds to lose and I had counted calories for over fifty years. Only you can make the "free-carbs" versus "limited-carbs" choice for yourself. I suggest trying intermittent fasting without restricting carbs at first to see how you do.

I decided to combine intermittent fasting with a LCHF diet to achieve results. This chapter is dedicated to people, like me, who are following a LCHF diet while on intermittent fasting.

What is a Ketogenic (Keto) diet?
1. A Keto diet is a low-carbohydrate, high-fat, moderate-protein diet which helps many to burn fat stores more easily. It is considered ultra-low carb and is not for everyone.
2. The goal of any LCHF diet is to force the body to burn fat easily.
3. Keto diets, the ultra-low carb diets, are low-carbohydrate (5% of daily calories), moderate-protein (20%), and high-fat (75%) diets. Check with a medical provider who knows your history before embarking on a LCHF diet.
4. Ketone bodies may be detected in breath, urine, and blood, when we switch to burning fat. You will see information about measuring ketone bodies in LCHF literature. You do not need to measure ketones but for more information, visit https://www.dietdoctor.com/need-check-ketones.
5. Urine Keto Sticks are simple and cheap. They measure acetoacetate in the urine (a ketone body.) I purchased them at www.amazon.com and used them for the first month of my LCHF journey because I love data. Did I need to do this? No. When we are in ketosis for a while, we get efficient at using ketones for fuel and don't excrete as much in the urine. The sticks, therefore, can provide false negatives. Ketone breath

meters are available, as well as blood ketone meters if you want to gather additional data on yourself. Refer to dietdoc-tor.com for more information. My personal thought is that you do not need them.

Frequently Asked Questions

1. Is the Ketogenic diet the same as the Atkins diet?
   Keto is similar to the Atkins diet. A major difference is that the Atkins diet mainly focused on lowering carbohydrates and not on specific macronutrient ratios.
2. Is it safe to follow a LCHF diet?
   Consult with a qualified healthcare provider who knows your medical history prior to embarking on a change in diet or fitness plan, especially if you have type 1 or type 2 diabetes, heart disease, are pregnant, trying to conceive, are breastfeeding, have adrenal fatigue, or have other medical conditions described above.
3. What are macronutrients and do I need to count them?
   Macronutrients (macros) are carbohydrates, protein, and fat. Google any Ketogenic calculator for specific macros if you wish to restrict carbs. Check out https://www.ruled.me/keto-calculator.
   This calculator is simple to use. Enter your gender, height, weight, age, body fat percentage, activity level, end goals, and how many grams of carbohydrates and protein you wish to eat on a daily basis. You will be provided with the macronutrients that are right for you.
4. What are net carbohydrates (carbs) versus total carbohydrates and what do experts say I should I count?
   Net carbohydrates are total carbohydrates minus fiber and sugar alcohols. Some of us (like me) are affected by

tiny amounts of carbohydrates. Net carbohydrates give us the "feeling" that we can enjoy higher carbs without consequences.

Jeff S. Volek, PhD, RD, and Stephen D. Phinney, MD, PhD, suggest "50 grams of total carbs a day is enough to induce nutritional ketosis," (http://ketofitnow.com/total-carbs-vs-net-carbs).

The right amount of carb intake is individualized. This is based on your own level of carbohydrate tolerance. For the first year of my IF journey, I stayed at 20 total carb grams daily or below. This is ultra-low-carb based on my severe calorie restrictions, as well as needing to drop over 100 pounds. You may not need this ultra-low carb restriction.

5. How do I determine my own carbohydrate tolerance?

    You are your own study of one and I cannot answer that for you. Severely overweight, overly dieted people (like me) can be quite sensitive to carbs. Younger people who wish to lose smaller amounts of weight might not be carb sensitive. I did not achieve weight loss until I limited my carbohydrates. Other folks have bodies that thrive on carbs. Many of you reading this book will not need to restrict carbs on your intermittent fasting plan. The only way to tell is to experiment.

LCHF tips I learned were to start the journey slowly. Don't dive intoa 24 hour fast on the first day. I began at 16 hours fasted and an 8 hour window. After a month on 16:8, I added thirty minutes to my daily fast. When I reached 23:1, that worked well for me. I was not losing as I needed to but remained patient for 6 weeks. At week 6, I began restricting carbs. Bingo, the weight fell off like our grandsons slide down a playground slide. Finally...my study of one was yielding results. Carbs were stalling me.

6. What are examples of foods containing higher amounts of carbohydrates if I choose to restrict them?

   Breads, grains, starchy vegetables, beer, pasta, juice ,soda, fruits, cereal, sweetened yogurt, low-fat and fat-free dairy products, beans, legumes, some sauces, alcohol, chips, crackers, honey, milk, baked goods, donuts, candy, and more.

7. What are examples of foods that are considered lower in carbohydrates?

   Meat (the fattier the better), chicken with the skin, fatty fish like salmon, butter, heavy cream, coconut oil, olive oil, eggs, vegetables such as (broccoli, cabbage, Brussels sprouts, cauliflower, kale, spinach, asparagus, zucchini, mushrooms, cucumbers, lettuce, avocados, onions, tomatoes, radishes, peppers, lettuce), full-fat cheeses, full-fat butters and creams (avoid regular and reduced-fat milk, cheeses, and creams as they contain milk sugar), nuts, and berries in moderation.

8. I enjoy social gatherings. Can I drink alcohol on IF?

   Of course you can (if alcohol has not been restricted for another reason). This is life so let's set ourselves up for long-term success. Vodka, whiskey, brandy (not fruity), gin, and tequila, are great options alone. The sugary additives and mixers add the carbs. Club soda is a great mixer. Low-carbohydrate wines are available in many wine specialty stores as well. They are amazingly tasty choices. I'm a huge fan of *Fit Vine Wines* and the Sauvignon Blanc is my personal favorite. Check out (www.fitvinewine.com).

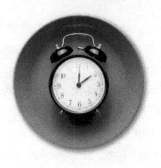

Chapter Eleven
How Do I Get Started?

*B*y this point of the book, something should be evident. If the low-fat, calorie-counting, increase your exercise, advice has been right, why are we getting fatter? Why do many of us dread January 2nd? How come so many Mondays equal "here we go again" days? Why did you buy another weight loss book? By the way, thank you!!

People lose weight counting, measuring, and buying low taste Frankenfoods. I did and I'm sure you have as well. They work on growing their grit and building their self-discipline muscles. They feel proud and committed to lose 5, 10, 20, 50, or even 100 pounds or more. They work hard and make sacrifices. They get thinner in the short-term. They swear by their diet plans because they are familiar like old sweatshirts. They think those of us who fast are crazy fad dieters. Heck, they have started that same diet on literally hundreds of Mondays. They know that those tasteless deli rounds with fat-free mayo and turkey are devoted to the goal. They convince themselves that low-fat yogurt makes them feel like they are behaving. They feel they are on solid ground when they order a salad, instead of a double cheeseburger. Oh...and they have dressing on the side....of the taco chips and croutons that is. It's just a salad, right? Do you see yourselves like I see myself? You bet you do. Remember my fried veggie bar days at work? Come on, it's just veggies...it's just salad...this deli flat and tasteless mayo doesn't taste that bad...

But then, there are dinner plans with family at a restaurant. The big "cheat" is a go. We are starving from all that fat-free mayo and we deserve it. After all, we have been dieting for two weeks and need a good meal. That cheat tastes so good. Amazing in fact! Bread is not tasteless and stale nothingness. Fat-free mayo is replaced by the parmesan special with extra cheese. Dessert is included so why not cherish that "free" chocolate cake? "I already cheated so when I get home....maybe a bowl of ice cream would be good to wash it all down. I only ate half of my cake." That turns into, "I might as well cheat all weekend and restart my deprivation on Monday." "No, we are going away in a month. I think I will resume my starvation on January 2nd." I am pretty sure that many people reading this think I know them. I get it guys. I get it.

So.....if this counting strategy worked well, why do we need to "sign up" again on January 2nd, on Monday after vacation, or before the next vacation or class reunion? Why are most dieters repeat customers? Failed long-term success yields higher profit margins. Fail guys....then come back for more deprivation...because it's comfortable. Ugh! Sound like you? It's evil and it's false marketing. I, for one, gave up more times than the gray hair on my head.

Why are 2/3 of Americans obese or overweight? Why is that curve climbing like our waistlines? Because losing weight by restricting calories is not the long-term solution. Being a sugar burner will not get you to where you want to be long-term. Face reality-it just will not.

Your problem has never been your commitment. The low-calorie deli rounds taste fake. Most frozen yogurt tastes good because the fat is replaced with sugar. Stop lowering your metabolism by counting calories. STOP! Stop looking at celebrities telling you to count! Seriously, if it works so well, how do you think their business models project increased revenue?

Stop thinking if you exercise twice a day, you can eat anything you want. You cannot exercise away bad food choices. We are not wired to outsmart our forks. Yes, exercise is important for overall health. No, exercise does not counteract a bad diet.

Find your hidden Jennifer Lopez, Ben Affleck, Beyonce, Christian Bale, Terry Crews, Hugh Jackman, Nicole Kidman, Benedict Cumberbatch, Liv Tyler, or Jimmy Kimmel. Intermittent fasting has been in the celeb circle for years and these folks are reportedly successful timekeepers too.

Do intermittent fasting, either with carb restriction or alone. Start being your own best timekeeper. Surrender your calorie counting. The past diet "experts" got it wrong.

Time to establish your goals.

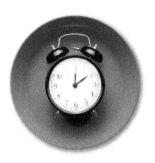

Chapter Twelve

Goals

*T*his is the most significant chapter in the book. You have the material, you have read my story, but how do you overcome your years of diet deficiency?

By getting your head in the game. You did not buy this book to read another self-help diet guide. If you did, you wasted your money. You bought this book because you are fed up with failing at diets. You're tired of feeling ashamed that you are overweight. You have maxed out on diet starts on Mondays. You are jaded by counting, losing, and regaining. Time to get your head into the right space.

- Think about the long-term impact of the healthier YOU.
- Visualize that healthy YOU. See it. Etch it firmly in your brain.
- Think about the lifelong impact of your new healthful life.
- Brainstorm with yourself. Think long and hard about why YOU want this.
- Why do you want a healthier life? Why do you want to lose weight?
- Set long-term goals and short-term goals.

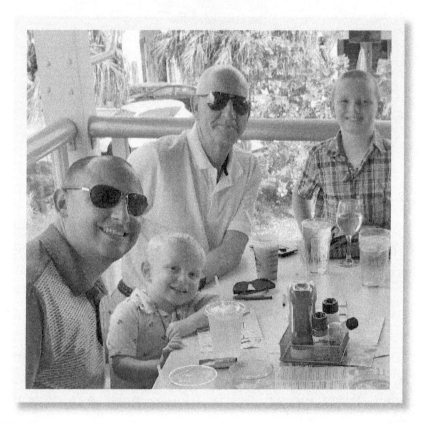

My main incentive: son Mike, grandson Ryan,
husband Marcel, grandson Lucas.

- ⏲ Make goals realistic for you. I will never wear a size zero-it's a fact. Setting that as a goal for me would be unrealistic.
- ⏲ Examine goals continually along your journey.
- ⏲ Be prepared to adjust. Life is never perfect. Be flexible.
- ⏲ Allow for occasional setbacks….they happen so move on.
- ⏲ Track successes beyond watching the scale. (I track photos and body measurements).

My Long-Term Goal

I will lead a healthy lifestyle by intermittently fasting, losing weight, and reducing my risks from weight-related conditions.

My major incentive is the value I hold for my husband, son, grandsons, family, and close friends. Being overweight put me at risk for a myriad of illnesses. I deserve to be flourishing with health as we all do. I need to be the best version of me to support myself, and to ultimately champion for them.

Achieving health is more compelling than a smaller pant size (although dropping six pant sizes has been sweet). So does that mean I will never eat cheesecake again? Heck no. This is my life, not a denial plan. When that turtle cheesecake is on the table, I reflect on if it's "worthy" before I devour it.

Stop, pause, and contemplate the long-term goal. In five minutes, the cheesecake will be finished. Bravo, a hit of sugar you thought you could not live without. Stop, pause, contemplate the long-term goal. Visualize the healthier version of you. For me, five minutes of cheesecake decadence no longer triumphs over the visualization of a healthier me.

There are times when I plan to eat that cheesecake. There is no guilt associated with planning food extravagances. Life happens and we can plan for splurges with no remorse. No need to jump off the wagon for the weekend and dread the following Monday diet restart.

On Thanksgiving, I enjoy stuffing (made with bread), mashed potatoes, and of course rolls. Being of Italian heritage, crispy pepper biscuits always signified Thanksgiving. These are planned treats and they are worth the indulgence. Here is the difference—I'm back on my plan the following morning. My timekeeper allows me to enjoy in my window, but go right back into fasting to reduce those glycogen stores. This translates into a sound relationship with food. Food is delicious and it fuels us. Make peace with that. It should not be our source of comfort or self-soothing. That ice cream sundae is not going to solve your boredom or your stressors.

Short-Term Goals

These goals should be measurable, attainable, and action-oriented.

I recommend setting at least three short-term goals or "mini goals."

Make them realistic, examine them frequently, tweak them as necessary, allow for setbacks, and for goodness sakes, celebrate victories without food rewards.

My own short-term or "mini goals"

1. I will lose the first fifteen pounds in three months.
2. I will lose 100 pounds by the conclusion of year two of my plan (averaging).
3. I will perform high-impact-interval-training in two of my weekly workouts. I will incorporate yoga within 6 months.
4. I will obtain baseline measurements of my waist, hips, arms, and legs, and will measure my monthly progress. Trust me,

when the scale stalls, these measurements are important. Would you believe that my waistline has dropped 18 inches? Yikes, no wonder the seatbelt on the plane is large.

5. I will end my scale obsession. There, I admit it. I am a recovering scale addict. Let me take off my earrings before I check my weight...ugh!

6. I will check my weight first thing in the morning for the first three months. Following that, I will weigh monthly. I have learned that weight loss is not linear. You can be the best faster on the planet, but weight changes occur due to salt, carbohydrates, exercise, weight of the food, medications, hormones, alcohol intake, etc. Overly obsessing on the scale is a big fat mistake. Many people weigh daily, but average weekly for a true weight picture.

7. I will take baseline pictures, and will take a facial selfie once a week. Taking selfies, while carrying excess pounds, is unpleasant. Trust me, it is worth the initial agony as you see the comparisons and view your progress.

8. I will participate in online Facebook fellowship support groups through social media. This provides support from like-minded people. I will support others in an empathic manner. This is a game changer people.

    My favorite Facebook support groups are *One Meal A Day IF Lifestyle*, and *Delay, Don't Deny: Intermittent* Fasting *Support*. These groups are the creation of Gin Stephens, author of *Delay, Don't Deny, and Feast Without Fear.* Both groups have a combined membership of over 100,000 worldwide members. They are closed groups with required entry questions. People outside of the groups cannot see your information. I strongly encourage you to check these groups out.

9. I will celebrate ten-pound losses with non-food rewards. Some

of my rewards have been a new top, a trendy nail polish, a latest book, etc. The greatest feeling is to downsize my jeans. I have done that six times so far. Overwhelmingly astounding!

10. I will memorialize fifty pound losses with a handbag. Anyone that knows me is aware of my love for handbags. Check out www.brahmin.com. The craftsmanship goes hand-in-hand with the tremendous efforts embedded within a fifty-pound weight loss. I have acquired two gorgeous handbags to date, by the way.

11. I will share non-scale victories (NSV's in the weight loss world) to encourage others. Some NSV's that I have discovered as a result of losing 100 pounds are:

   a. Blood lipid panel better than desirable range.
   b. Blood glucose no longer prediabetic.
   c. High blood pressure gone.
   d. Esophageal reflux gone.
   e. Arthritic aches and pains gone.
   f. Incredible energy and mental focus profound.
   g. Skin tags disappeared on their own.
   h. Thick, red, inch-wide scar from a prior surgery gone!!
   i. Theater seats are huge. Anyone overweight gets this.
   j. Airplane seats are comfortable. Yes, it's true!
   k. Seatbelts on the plane have a ten inch surplus.
   l. Seating in restaurants is comfortable. Life in a normally sized body is just plain victorious!

In summary, develop a long-term goal that is your main motivation. Brainstorm with yourself to develop "mini-goals" that are real, measurable, never perfect, and celebrated along the way. Participate in fellowship support groups so you are surrounded by like-minded people. Lastly, believe that nothing on that fork will ever be more valuable than reaching your goals. You are so worth it.

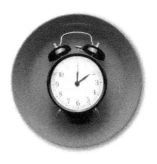

Chapter Thirteen
What Can I Eat On IF?

*D*rumroll........**if you choose intermittent fasting with no carbohydrate restriction,** eat whatever you want within your window. Congratulations, dietary freedom has arrived. Check your guilt at the curb. Fuel your body with nutritious items. Pay attention to the quality of your choices. Remember that IF is not a license to eat junk food to excess. Every reasonable thinking person knows that already. Enough said.

1. Choose the times to fast and times to eat. You are officially on your way to becoming a fat burner. Welcome to the club.
2. A great starting point is 16:8. In the IF world, that means 16 fasted hours with an 8 hour window. 16:8 is a great way to ease into your fasting lifestyle.
3. A popular version of 16:8 is **fasting** from 8pm-12 noon because many of us sleep through most of those hours.
4. A typical **eating window** on 16:8 is 12 noon-8pm. That means you enjoy food between 12 noon and 8 pm. This is how many of us start the IF journey. Get your timekeeper ready to go.

5. During the fast, keep it pure. Pure fasts help us to become fat burners more quickly. Abandon your belief that eating frequently "keeps up your metabolism." Eating produces insulin. The more frequently we eat, the more we produce insulin, the harder it is to gobble up your body fat.

6. What can I have during the pure fast on IF?
    - 🕐 Black unflavored coffee (I know, it sounds impossible)
    - 🕐 Water
    - 🕐 Unflavored sparkling water
    - 🕐 Unflavored tea
        - ⊘ No diet drinks or diet soda...stop that diet soda ASAP.
        - ⊘ No flavored coffee beans
        - ⊘ No fruity water drops
        - ⊘ No low-calorie, low-fat creamers
        - ⊘ No artificial sweeteners even though they have zero calories. They do spike insulin which slows fat burning.
        - ⊘ No mints, candies, or sugarless gum. Each time your body senses something sweet it produces insulin.

7. What can I eat in my 8 hour eating window?
    An 8 hour window could include two meals and one snack.
    An 8 hour window could include a snack, one meal, and a dessert.
    An 8 hour window could include two snacks and one meal.

You get the picture. The eating window is what you want it to be. It's flexible. Deliciousness 101.

8. Should I count calories in my eating window? There are a lot of conflicting views on this in the IF literature.

I do not suggest calorie counting. All calories are not created equally. Restricting calories forces our bodies to work slower to match the lower intake. How has that worked for us in the past?

Check out Dr. Fung's view at, https://idmprogram.com/difference-calorie-restriction-fasting-fasting-27.

Smart choices are whole, nutrient-dense foods, not prepackaged foods. Do not fear healthy fats! I will say that again, do not fear healthy fats! Foods that are nutrient-rich are great options. A package of donuts is never superior to a plate of fresh vegetables. Listen to your body.

9. Should I count macronutrients in my window to follow IF? It sounds complicated and overwhelming.

   If you are not restricting carbs, do not worry about macros. You are free to eat foods that fuel your body well. My advice is to try IF alone to see if you achieve success. That might be all you need. Many suggest restricting carbs first and then adding IF. It is your choice. The logic behind that is when you first follow a LCHF diet, you become a fat burner faster making IF easier to follow. Intermittent fasting is not a one-size-fits-all plan.

   If you are doing IF and restricting carbs like me, then yes, you need to count macros. I was not one of the lucky ones. For me, LCHF was simple and I never felt deprived.

10. What is a macronutrient "macro"?

    Food consists of three macros:
    - ⏱ Carbohydrates
    - ⏱ Proteins
    - ⏱ Fats

11. If you are doing intermittent fasting along with LCHF, here is a suggested start:

    Find a ketogenic calculator online. There are many available.

    - Enter metric or imperial units (imperial in the US).
    - Enter your gender.
    - Add height and weight.
    - Enter your age.
    - Enter your body fat percentage. There is a visual guide to help you to determine that.
    - Record your activity level.
    - List your goals (there are prompts to help).
    - Enter the carbohydrates you want to consume daily.
    - Add the amount of protein you need based on activity. The calculator will then reveal your macronutrient ratio.

My favorite calculator is found at www.ruledme.com.

    - Get yourself a food scale. I paid $15.00 for an Ozeri Pro Digital Kitchen Scale from www.amazon.com. When you count macros, visual estimates can be inaccurate. My idea of a one ounce portion of macadamia nuts was a four ounce portion.

12. What are examples of foods to eat on IF along with a LCHF diet?

    - Eggs are a staple. They are delicious fried in butter and oil.
    - Fish with no breading is fabulous. Fattier fish like salmon is a staple on my diet.
    - Vegetables that grow above ground are good options (fresh or frozen) zucchini, lettuce, mushrooms,

cucumbers, radishes olives, peppers, cauliflower (list just a sampling).

- ☺ Nuts (watch portions as nuts can be trigger foods to overeat). I measure one to two ounces on my food scale and avoid cashews as they are higher in carbohydrates.

- ☺ Meats, the fattier the better. On a keto diet, fat is your friend. Eating fat helps to burn your own fat. Yes, that is not a typo. Eat the fat baby! I love to cook in butter, olive oil, and/or coconut oil. Avoid ketchup on keto as it loaded with sugar.

- ☺ High-fat dairy products are mainstays. Butter, full-fat yogurt, heavy cream, sour cream, full-fat cheeses are key. Stay away from dairy that is light or low-fat as it contains more sugar.

- ☺ Berries in moderation with heavy cream are a treat! Raspberries and blackberries are the best options on Keto.

13. What are examples of foods to consider as snacks (both on IF and on LCHF)?

- ☺ Cheese
- ☺ Avocado
- ☺ Olives
- ☺ Nut butters
- ☺ Bacon and pepperoni
- ☺ Nuts (macadamia nuts are the lowest in carbohydrates)
- ☺ Eggs
- ☺ Cheese crisps
- ☺ Cut up veggie sticks dipped in cream cheese
- ☺ Berries (raspberries and blackberries are the most keto friendly)

- ⏱ A few squares of 70 to 85% chocolate
- ⏱ Low carb zucchini chips (yum)

14. What to avoid if you are following LCHF?
- ⊘ Candy
- ⊘ Soda/Fruit Juice
- ⊘ Beer/Sweet Cocktails
- ⊘ Potatoes/Rice/Pasta
- ⊘ Many Fruits
- ⊘ Bread
- ⊘ Donuts

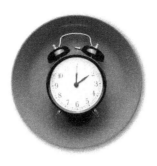

Chapter Fourteen

Eating Out/Vacations

*E*ating out on IF is part of life. Plan social gatherings within your window, if you can. Our grandson, Lucas, tells servers, "New Nana does not eat in the morning. She has an evening window." If that is not possible, be flexible with your window. Life happens and you are more apt to make this a lifestyle when you are not rigid. Restaurant meals, when eating a low-carb diet, have many available options. Here are some low-carb dining tips. These pointers also apply if you're doing intermittent fasting and not restricting carbs.

1. Eat a fatty snack before you leave home. Check the menu ahead if you can. It's easier to make your meal plan first without the social distractions. Olives, cheese, or nuts are great snacks to stall off hunger before you leave home.
2. Avoid buffets. If you find yourself with no other option, skip the breads, grains, potatoes, and sugary treats. Fill up on fats, vegetables, and sparingly on proteins. Be careful with sauces and gravies as many contain hidden sugars.
3. At a burger/sandwich place, order the protein on lettuce

with no roll. Load your plate with vegetables and avoid ketchup and barbecue sauces as they are high in sugar. Skip the fries and ask for mushrooms or sliced tomatoes.

4. At an Asian or Chinese restaurant, stir-fry dishes without rice are great selections. Skip the sweet and sour dishes and battered appetizers. Egg Foo Young without brown gravy is also a great low-carb idea. I always get shrimp Egg Foo Young.

5. At a Mexican restaurant, pass on the beans, tortilla chips, and rice. Try the protein mixed with cheese, sour cream, guacamole, and vegetables. I order shrimp fajitas and leave the tortillas. I enjoy salsa but ask for fresh veggies to replace the chips. I have never found a Mexican restaurant that cannot make a plate of cucumbers, tomatoes, celery, and carrots.

6. At a pizza restaurant, salads with meats and cheeses are alternatives. If you are craving pizza, order it with cheese, meats, and the vegetable toppings you love. Just scrape off the toppings and leave the crust behind. I promise, it still can be delicious.

7. At breakfast places and cafes, eggs and meats are good votes. Skip the pancakes, syrups, toast, and bagels.

8. Vacations, while enjoyable, for dieters, can pack anxiety into that suitcase. Do not be anxious about your intermittent fasting lifestyle on vacation.

    a. Realize that IF is a lifestyle. Food and drink on vacation are parts of the experience. Enjoy the flavors without guilt or shame.

    b. Prepare to be flexible with your window. Fast as long as you can each day. Don't worry if your window is longer than it usually is. Big deal. It all balances out.

    c. Eat what and when you decide to eat, not when others make you feel you have to. If your group goes out for breakfast, sip your black coffee or tea. Enjoy their company without the maple syrup if that is your choice. Open your window when your inner timekeeper says YOU want to.

d. Enjoy cocktails but watch the mixers. I found that *Fit Vine Wine* (www.fitvinewine.com), and vodka martinis with extra olives, are great selections. Please note that alcoholic beverages "pack a punch" when you fast. A few nuts, veggies, or cheese before that drink can be most helpful.

e. Be assertive and ask servers for your special dietary requests.

f. Most restaurants are more than willing to accommodate.

g. We have cruised twice on intermittent fasting. I was anxious about the food. Don't be! Relax! Cruise vacations make IF and LCHF simple. There are numerous food options so staying on your plan is actually simple.

Vacation/cruise tips: Grab items you want from the ship and store them in your room until your window opens. At dinner, tell the server if you eat a LCHF diet. They will accommodate. On our last two week cruise, since my window is an evening window, I went to breakfast and lunch but sipped black coffee. I took bacon, cheese, olives, and fresh veggies, to our cabin. I opened my window before dinner with a cocktail and my room treats. At dinner, I asked the server for double veggies to replace potatoes and rice. There were plenty of LCHF desserts and they were all heavenly. When I returned home, I had actually lost weight. Eat on vacation when it's right for you. Don't eat because you feel pressured by others.

If you decide to overly indulge while on vacation, enjoy your decision. The benefit to intermittent fasting is that there should be no guilt or self-blame attached to indulgences.

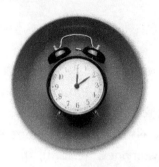

Chapter Fifteen
Eat That Treat

Intermittent fasting is a manner of living. There will be times when you will eat those treats and indulgences. There will be foods that are served in your homes or at your favorite restaurants that you decide to enjoy. Go for it. Here are some common diet derailing scenarios that might occur:

- ⏰ You have a night window and there is a special brunch at work.
- ⏰ Your Nana bakes monkey bread and you feel badly refusing.
- ⏰ You join colleagues at a café and the toasted sesame bagel smells divine. It's all you can think of.

You get the picture. Lose the guilt and the drop the shame. It does not fit into this lifestyle. Be kind and embrace yourself. Ease up on the perfection pedal. This is our life and there will be good reasons we choose to deviate from our plans. Calling the enjoyment of foods, "cheating," does not fit into this lifestyle.

Tips:

1. Make the choice to eat off plan when the food is worth it.
2. Cheating projects a negative message. I prefer to say I plan worthy treats.
3. Never eat because someone expects you to.
4. Do not strive for diet perfection. This is a journey and we are human.
5. Every time you see good food, it is not a free pass to indulge.
6. Weekends are not holidays.
7. Set the long-term goal of better health in your brain.
8. Before you decide if a treat is worthy, pause and remind yourself of the goals.
9. When a food indulgence is planned, enjoy food that is worthy.
10. Treat yourself with foods that have sufficient fats to keep insulin spikes low. The slice of bread is small but the slather of butter is abundant.
11. Don't turn to food to provide comfort. That becomes a vicious cycle.
12. Don't blame yourself following a treat. Learn from how it impacted your body, and jump back on the plan. No more restart Mondays.

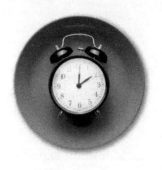

Chapter Sixteen
The Pesky Plateau

Weight loss plateaus (stalls) are commonplace. Don't panic. We all have them. Remember that weight loss is never linear. There are numerous factors that impact that number on the scale. We are works in progress and a true plateau is a stall for three to six weeks or more. I know, I wanted to lose ten pounds overnight too.

What can you do to push through a plateau?

1. Take a look at what you are eating. Reassess your habits. Look at your salt intake and possible water retention. Do not throw in the towel. You may be eating more food than your body needs. When you eat, stop when you're comfortable but not overly stuffed. Listen to your body's satiety signals.

2. Is there a food sensitivity you might have? For me, more than two ounces of cheese stalls my progress. My own visual estimate of one ounce of nuts was actually four ounces.

3. Are you getting enough sleep? Lack of proper sleep can hinder weight loss.

4. Are you exercising too much? Your body can actually slow weight loss in response to too much exercise. Allow

yourself a recovery period.

5. Is your body in the adjustment phase? There are instances where your body replaces lost fat with water (sort of a place holder). All of a sudden, you experience the "whoosh." The extra water is released and a person can shed as much as five pounds in two days. We love the whoosh.

6. Stress can slow your weight loss by the production of the hormone cortisol. Stress reduction can increase weight loss.

7. If you are not restricting carbs, trying a low-carb diet for a few weeks might make it easier to feel full longer and break the plateau.

8. Alcohol might be stalling you (sorry all). Alcohol can interfere with weight loss because it is empty calories.

9. Your plateau may only be on the scale. In intermittent fasting, your body can be getting leaner but your weight is stuck. Check your body measurements, pictures, and the fit of your clothing for a true assessment. My pants fall off often when the scale is stagnant.

10. There is nothing wrong with planned indulgences. If you plan a treat, do it with no guilt. Hop right back on the journey. Don't make a planned treat a month-long derailment.

11. Check your comparison photos. A pound of muscle takes up less body space than a pound of fat. Check to see how those jeans are fitting. Trust me on this one.

12. You have a goal weight number in your head but it may not be realistic. Are you dreaming of a number that is beyond your set-point?

13. Keep your body guessing. Switch your window timing for a few days. Rotate your routine. You get the picture—shake things up.

14. Focus on the quality of your foods. While you might have had success eating cake in your window, it might be time to

focus on eliminating sugary processed foods. Increase the quality of your whole foods to get through the plateau.

Pesky plateau tips—Strength training by lifting weights has allowed me to lose body fat. I drink at least 100 ounces of water daily to lessen my cravings and reduce my over-eating. Do not cut calories to ramp up your weight loss. It does not work. Beware of mindless snacking because you think the snacks are healthy. For me, trigger foods are nuts and cheese. When I hit my plateau, I went back to measuring my nut portions (1 ounce), and my cheese portions (2 ounces). That, coupled with additional strength training, pushed through my plateaus. I have also added a few 48 hour fasts when the scale hits a stone wall. Whatever you do, know that each step forward is in the right direction.

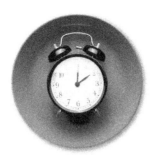

Chapter Seventeen

Hunger Is Not A Game

*P*erhaps by this point in the book, you may have a fear of hunger. Many of us feared hunger when we first learned about intermittent fasting. News flash-hunger is learned and we can survive it. Intermittent fasting does not induce extreme hunger that is followed by binge eating. That happened in our rice cake era, not with intermittent fasting.

Hunger typically begins four to eight hours after we close our windows. Fasting actually lessens our hunger sensations. How does that happen?

1. Hunger is a learned response.
2. Hunger happens in waves. Ride the waves by keeping busy.
3. Hunger is patterned to follow certain times of the day when we eat three meals and snacks. Hunger occurs before those meals because it is a normal response to an expectation.
4. Hunger is often paired with events like football games or movies.
5. Intermittent fasting breaks the patterns and expectations of food every few hours.

6. Intermittent fasting serves to reduce overall hunger.
7. Eat when your hunger results in dizziness and the inability to function in your life.

Hunger tips—I have learned that hunger is usually associated with my not having sufficient healthy fats during my OMAD. I combat hunger by drinking water, sparkling water, or black coffee. Keeping busy is the best way to ride that hunger wave. My closets have never been more organized!

As an aside, speaking of closet organization, make the decision to ditch the big clothes. Do not let them linger in your closet as security. Hopefully, some large-sized women purchased my donated suits, coats, and pants, for very reasonable prices at the donation center. And don't buy a new wardrobe with each smaller size. Those pant sizes drop quickly on intermittent fasting.

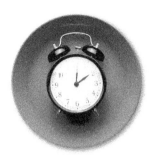

Chapter Eighteen

Coffee/Tea, Smoothies, and Energy Bars

These topics are scattered throughout intermittent fasting literature and warrant a mention:

1. Coffee/Tea
    - ⏱ Coffee/tea is important for many people (like me).
    - ⏱ Coffee/tea is not required for intermittent fasting.
    - ⏱ During the pure fast-black coffee/tea matters. No milk, no creamers, no sweeteners. You can adjust.
    - ⏱ Black coffee/tea does not break your fast.
    - ⏱ Avoid flavored coffee beans and flavored teas, as they do spike insulin.
    - ⏱ Coffee/tea has appetite suppressing effects and can be helpful in weight loss.
    - ⏱ Coffee/tea can increase energy and cognitive function.
    - ⏱ Coffee/tea can promote autophagy (cellular repair).
    - ⏱ Yes-you can get used to black coffee and tea. You can-honest! A packet of Stevia or a splash of cream will stall your pure fast Don't do it. It took me a full

year not to dislike black coffee. Now, it's enjoyable.

⏱ You will see conflicting information regarding adding cream and sweetener to coffee/tea. Why chance undermining your pure fast?

⏱ "Bulletproof" coffee is loved by many fasters. You will see it referenced in IF literature. Bulletproof coffee is believed to enhance metabolism. It is coffee with butter/oil added, as well as Medium Chain Triglycerides (MCTs). It is not necessary and should never be consumed during the fast.

2. Smoothies-are they healthy?

    ⏱ Smoothies can be helpful if you control the ingredients.

    ⏱ Smoothies can be used for detox purposes, as well as for weight loss.

    ⏱ Smoothies should contain nutrient-rich ingredients.

    ⏱ Leafy vegetables, avocado, berries, greens, chia seeds, honey, nuts, and organic yogurt, are wonderful components for smoothies.

    ⏱ Avoid fruit juices, canned fruits, and extra added sugar.

    ⏱ While smoothies can be nutritious and satiating, be certain you allow room for the rest of the nutrients your body requires.

3. Energy Bars-are they healthy?

    ⏱ We have all seen energy bars in the stores. They are everywhere-in the diet aisle, in the breakfast food aisle, in the sports section, etc.

    ⏱ Bars can be helpful and tasty but they are not required for intermittent fasting.

    ⏱ Energy bars have their place and can serve as a holdover for days when life stalls the opening of the

eating window.
- 🕐 Energy bars can be purchased or can be made at home.

These are bars that I have tried:

- 🕐 *Quest Bars* are low-carb friendly and can be a good source of protein and fat.
- 🕐 *Perfect Bars* are organic, kosher, preservative-free, natural bars that are packed with nutrients. They are stored in the refrigerator section. Honey is the only added sweetener and they are the hottest trend in energy bars. These are my personal favorite.
- 🕐 *Kind Bars* contain delicious ingredients, are great sources of fiber, and have a low glycemic index. The lower the glycemic index, the less impact the bar has on blood sugar production.

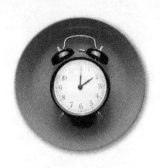

Chapter Nineteen
Artificial Sweeteners

A rtificial sweeteners deserve their own chapter as they are discussed heavily in the intermittent fasting community. Artificial sweeteners are synthetic sugar substitutes. According to Cleveland Clinic, the best artificial sweetener is no artificial sweetener.

In order to reap the benefits of weight loss and improved health from intermittent fasting, fasted hours must remain pure. While artificial sweeteners do not contain calories, they do provoke an insulin response as our body senses something sweet. All sweeteners have potentially negative effects on fasting. It is best to avoid them. If you need something sweet within your eating window, check out:

https://www.dietdoctor.com/low-carb/sweeteners.

To summarize the review by Diet Doctor, Dr. Andreas Eenfeldt, MD,

- ⊕ All sweeteners have possible negative side effects.
- ⊕ While there are negatives to all sweeteners, *Stevia*, *Erythritol*, and *Xylitol* are better options.
- ⊕ *Stevia*-commonly known as sugar leaf, is herbal and does

not contain carbs or calories. It does, however, have a distinctive aftertaste.

- ⏱ *Erythritol* is a sugar alcohol and it occurs naturally in plants.
- ⏱ *Xylitol* is another sugar alcohol found in plants.
- ⏱ *Splenda, Equal, and Sweet' N Low* are not recommended because each packet contains 0.9 grams of carbohydrates.

As you can see, artificial sweeteners are not recommended in intermittent fasting lifestyles. It is always better to enjoy foods in their natural states. For additional reading, review IDM's Diet Soda Delusion at:

https://idmprogram.com/the-diet-soda-delusion-the-epiphe-nomenon-of-obesity.

Sweetener tip: Monk fruit sweetener is an Asian fruit that is a natural way to replace sugar. Monk fruit is quite popular in the keto community. It is made from fruit extract, has zero carbs, yet can be difficult to find in U.S. markets. Monk fruit is reported as being 300 times sweeter than sugar.

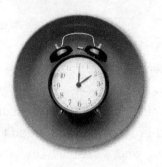

Chapter Twenty
Supplements/Medications

*D*ietary supplements/vitamins are often noted in literature on intermittent fasting. Supplements/vitamins are beyond the scope of this book. Based on your own health needs, the supplement/vitamin decision needs to be made jointly with your own healthcare provider.

The U.S. Food and Drug Administration (FDA) does not determine the effectiveness of dietary supplements/vitamins. Please refer to www.ods.od.nih.gov for more information. The National Institutes of Health (NIH) has prepared fact sheets regarding vitamins, minerals, and dietary supplements.

According to Dr. Jason Fung, few supplements are suggested,

https://medium.com/@drjasonfung/the-lack-of-benefits-of-supplements-65bc09eb9774.

Note the following supplements/vitamins that are seen frequently in the IF literature. I am not recommending the use or lack of use of these supplements/vitamins. These are listed for informational purposes:

1. Vitamin A-for vision, immune health, and organ health.
2. Branch-chain-amino acids(BCAAs)-for athletic performance.
3. Vitamin B complex-for multitude of uses.
4. Vitamin D-for stronger bones.
5. Electrolytes-Sodium and Potassium-for energy, fluid regulation, and charging the cells.
6. Fish oil/ Omega-3 Fatty Acids- for energy and organ function.
7. Magnesium-for muscle and nerve function. May reduce muscle cramping.
8. Probiotics-Live microorganisms intended for gut health benefits.
9. Turmeric-for reduction of inflammation.
10. Himalayan Pink Salt-contains 84 trace elements and is considered pure. You will see reference to sole (pronounced sole-ay) in IF literature. Sole is Himalayan Pink Salt in water. Since I started on a Keto diet, I use Himalayan Pink Salt daily. I place ¼ teaspoon under my tongue before my workout. I have never experienced a leg cramp since doing this.

Medications, on the other hand, that may or may not be part of your own health plan, cannot be overlooked. Any and all medications should be taken as prescribed.

Certain common medications may cause stomach upset and nausea if consumed on empty stomachs. Discuss medication management with your provider. If medications are necessary with food during your fasted hours, some people take them with a spoon of heavy cream, or with a leafy vegetable to maintain medication compliance and spike the least insulin response.

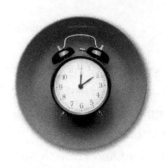

Chapter Twenty-One
Checklist to Start/Grocery List

Ok, so there has been a lot of information provided. You're willing to try. You're making the commitment to jump in. Your inner timekeeper is ready to roll.

I know for me, I gathered information, carefully reviewed it, and made the decision that I would begin. Now what? I was not quite sure how to best proceed. Are you overwhelmed? I certainly was. If you're like me, you want to keep life simple. While it was comforting to read that everyone fuels their bodies based on their own needs, what did that mean for me? I was used to eating tasteless food based on low calorie counts.

This chapter is dedicated to getting you started. It is not intended as the best plan to follow. It is proposed to make your new journey uncomplicated as you begin. Checklists help so let's review some important points:

Checklist to Start

1. Set your goals as we discussed in chapter 12. Goals are crucial for success and for continued motivation.

2. Review the exceptions to starting IF as identified in chapter 6. Discuss with your healthcare provider as indicated. Your safety is essential.

3. Discuss any changes in diet and health with your physician. Please do not take medical advice from people via the internet.

4. Eat dinner tonight as usual. You do not need to wait until Monday to start IF. Start now.

5. If you have chosen an evening window, you are done with food and drink for the day. Enjoy water, black unflavored coffee, or black tea, until you decide to open your window tomorrow. It's that simple. Ready, set, go....you're on the way.

6. Go to sleep and skip the popcorn and ice cream tonight.

7. Awaken and go about your normal routine in the morning.

8. Have no food or beverages when you awaken, other than water, black coffee, or plain tea. Remember the fast must be pure.

9. When your window opens, eat foods you enjoy. That's it.

10. You are now an intermittent faster. Yes, it is that simple.

Grocery List

The food freedom with intermittent fasting is amazing, yet frightening. Almost unbelievable in fact. On the flip side, there are foods you can include in your intermittent fasting life- but what are they? Remember, we are restricting hours, we are not restricting calories. So what can we eat? What should we include in our pre-intermittent fasting grocery haul? The following list helped me. This is a guide to get you started whether you are restricting carbs or not:

1. Water
   Unflavored
   Plain or sparkling
2. Vegetables
   Asparagus
   Broccoli
   Cauliflower
   Brussels sprouts
   Cabbage
   Celery
   Cucumbers
   Eggplant
   Lettuce
   Kale
   Mushrooms
   Spinach
   Radishes
   Zucchini
   Onions
   Peppers
   Tomatoes
3. Dairy
   Eggs
   Full-fat cheeses
   Heavy cream
   Sour cream
   Butter/Ghee
   Cream cheese
   Full-fat yogurt
   Crème Fraiche

4. Meats
    Bacon
    Ground beef
    Steak
    Chicken breasts and thighs
    Pork chops and pork tenderloin
    Ham
    Turkey
    Salami/Pepperoni
    Prosciutto
    Sausage
5. Seafood
    Salmon
    Cod
    Snapper
    Shrimp
    Scallops
    Cod
    Lobster
    Mussels
    Tuna
    Tilapia
    Crabmeat
    Clams
6. Fruits
    Blackberries
    Raspberries
    Strawberries
    Blueberries
    Avocados

7. Dressings/Condiments
    Mustard
    Olive oil
    Coconut oil
    Ketchup (reduced sugar)
    Full-fat salad dressings
8. Snacks
    Macadamia nuts
    Brazil nuts
    Pecans
    Peanuts
    Almonds
    Hazelnuts
    Olives
    Full-fat cheese sticks
    Guacamole
9. Miscellaneous
    Plain, unflavored coffee
    Plain, unflavored tea
    Peanut butter
    Nut butter (I love almond butter)
    Dark chocolate (minimum of 80% cacao)
    If you need sweeteners in your window, I prefer
    Swerve, and Monk Fruit
    Almond Flour (for the carb restricters)
    Unsweetened Cocoa (Trader Joe's is great)
    Coconut oil nonstick spray
    Full-fat mayonnaise

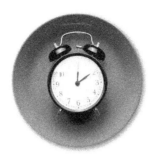

Chapter Twenty-Two
Sample OMAD Menus

We have established that intermittent fasting is an eating plan that restricts hours and not foods. Perhaps, you might need more guidance than a grocery list and the notion that the plan works if you listen to your body. What? My body? I'm not sure I know how to listen to my body just yet. Wasn't my body telling me to eat two donuts not that long ago?

In order to get started, I am sharing some of my favorite meals. Be reminded that I ate low-carbohydrate high-fat for my first year. You may be eating carbs more liberally than I did so tweak these as you wish. These menus are merely here as examples. I prefer to keep my intermittent fasting life simple. My guess is, you will also.

1. Cheese omelet (3 eggs) with 4 strips of cooked bacon
   Cucumber and tomato salad in 2 tablespoons olive oil
   6 large green stuffed olives (I love the ones stuffed with blue cheese)
   2 ounces Swiss cheese
   2 tablespoons Kerrygold Grass Fed butter
   1 cup sautéed zucchini in olive oil with shredded parmesan

2. 5 ounces grilled salmon
    1 cup grilled yellow squash
    ½ cup red bell peppers
    2 ounces cheddar cheese
    1 tablespoon sour cream
    2 tablespoons Kerrygold butter
    1 tablespoon organic almond butter
    4 sticks celery

3. 6 ounces stir-fried 85% ground beef in 2 tablespoons olive oil
    1 tablespoon onion
    2 ounces cheddar cheese
    ½ cup green beans
    5 large radishes
    2 tablespoons *Marie's Blue Cheese* (not light) dressing
    2 hard-boiled eggs
    2 stalks celery with peanut butter

4. 6 ounces stir-fried chicken breasts in 3 tablespoons olive oil
    5 ounces portobello mushrooms cooked in butter
    ½ avocado in olive oil
    1 cucumber in olive oil
    2 ounces pepper jack cheese
    5 green stuffed olives
    ½ cup green beans in 2 tablespoons butter
    2 ounces fresh mozzarella cheese
    Raspberries and heavy cream

5. Pan-fried sea scallops(6) in olive oil and butter
    Eggplant grilled with oil
    2 ounces Kerrygold Swiss cheese
    Radishes and tomato salad with blue cheese

2 ounces macadamia nuts
2 strips cooked bacon
2 hard-boiled eggs
½ cup ricotta cheese (whole-milk)

6. 2 grilled pork chops with mushrooms
Sautéed spinach and tomatoes cooked in Kerrygold butter
2 ounces of cheddar cheese
Radishes and cucumber salad with 2 tablespoons olive oil
Celery, almonds, and peanut butter
½ avocado in olive oil

7. Beef burrito in a bowl with no shell
Sour cream, lettuce, salsa, cheddar cheese
½ cup spaghetti squash with butter
Green olives
Raspberries, blueberries, and Crème Fraiche

During my window, coffee with heavy cream is a decadent treat.
While preparing dinner, I snack on macadamia nuts, almonds, or green olives.

For dessert, I love berries and heavy cream. If I crave chocolate, I enjoy a Keto Mug Cake https://www.ruled.me/keto-chocolate-cake-mug. I also adore Perfect Bars, https://perfectbar.com

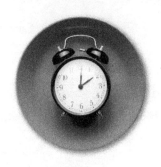

Chapter Twenty-Three
To Tell or Remain Silent

We live in an eating universe. Telling others about intermittent fasting versus keeping it to ourselves, is a common topic of discussion. Should we tell or remain silent?

It is 100% your call whether or not you tell others you are doing intermittent fasting. Let me share some of my **telling tips:**

1. I kept my journey quiet, other than to my husband, for the first three months. Marcel was my major supporter!

2. During the first three months, I said I had already eaten, or that I was not hungry. It worked well with little pushback from others.

3. Once I hit the three month point and had proven success, I shared IF when people asked. My weight loss was obvious at this point and I had secured my intermittent fasting confidence.

4. When asked, I described intermittent fasting. I told people I had thoroughly researched it, that it was scientifically sound, and that I had never felt better. I requested their support, rather than their criticism.

5. Be prepared for stares, dropped jaws, odd looks, rolling eyes, and these types of comments:
    - ⊘ You will slow your metabolism.
    - ⊘ You will gain it back when you quit the diet.
    - ⊘ I could never do that. I need breakfast.
    - ⊘ Aren't you afraid you will be hungry?
    - ⊘ It's unhealthy not to eat.
    - ⊘ You're on another diet fad?
    - ⊘ Your cholesterol numbers will go up with all that butter. I'm worried about my own cholesterol.
    - ⊘ You will lose muscle...blah...blah...blah.

6. Telling others can be positive or can create negativity. People may feel threatened about their own eating habits. They know how hard dieting can be. Change is difficult for those who are not ready. Some criticize intermittent fasting rather than admit that they don't have the faith in themselves to try. Many fear failure and I understand that.

7. Today, almost two years into my journey, I share intermittent fasting with everyone who has interest. I never criticize anyone's chosen weight loss plan and don't judge the foods on another's plate. I do, however, respond to those who ask about my own weight loss, as an empathic and caring educator.

8. It is a great pleasure to share this discovery with others who think calorie counting and exercise are their answers. I am passionate about intermittent fasting and am hopeful that the naysayers can open their minds to the premise that we have been lied to.

9. A great blog post to support the difference between intermittent fasting and the calorie restriction is listed in the IDM blog. Share this with the naysayers. I listed this post

previously in the book and am listing it again here due to its extreme significance. Thank you for this great story, Dr. Fung!

https://idmprogram.com/difference-calorie-restriction-fasting-fasting-27/.

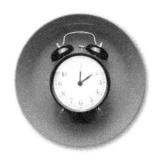

Chapter Twenty-Four
Inspiration

*M*otivation keeps us going when the going gets rough. We are human and there are ups and downs along the road. Here are some **inspirational tips** that have guided me along my own journey:

1. Be the best version of you that you can be. Let those goals drive you forward.
2. Train your brain that willpower is a skill you can master.
3. A goal with no action is words on a page.
4. Self-doubt kills progress more than failure.
5. If you slip, get up and keep going strong.
6. Success begins with your mind, not with the gym.
7. Break your old, conditioned responses to foods.
8. Hardwire healthier habits.
9. Push yourself because if you don't, nobody else will.
10. You can make a commitment to change.
11. Always remind yourself why you started. I do this daily.
12. Nobody is ever destined to be overweight. We can break the cycle.

13. Healthy and fit are better than anything on that plate. Anything!
14. The only failure is failing to try.
15. Get your inner timekeeper ready to guide you to rock this intermittent lifestyle.

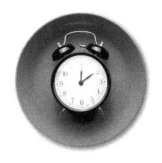

Chapter Twenty-Five
The Flip-Side

I debated about adding this final chapter. I am not in maintenance yet and am still working toward that goal. The reality is that once you lose a significant amount of weight, life changes. Let me share some changes you may experience as you move forward. It's helpful to be prepared.

Get ready to adjust to your life as a normally-sized person. You are approaching the finish line of your weight loss, or, you are simply making good progress. What then?

As I write this chapter, I have dropped over 100 pounds. I have lost an entire person. I am not driven by numbers on a chart. My goal is to keep losing weight until I feel that my body has reached its best set point. I'm not there yet.

Reflecting back on life carrying around an excessive hundred pounds is daunting. Many of us feel unattractive, unhealthy, exhausted, and that we don't fit into the healthy universe. Social situations are hard, travel is nearly impossible, and don't even get me started on how distressing it is to find fashionable clothing.

Now, you're well on your way to the slimmer you. You many be near the finish line, like me. Everything changes!

You're thinner, happier, free in your own skin, not winded when you move, your joints don't hurt from carrying the pounds, you have increased stamina, and you're confident because you feel better. You're proud that you are succeeding. Losing weight can be difficult and you're doing it on intermittent fasting. Give your all-star timekeeper a raise! Bravo!

Your life will not become perfect because you lost weight. Don't expect that. High-fives because you reduced your risk of obesity-related concerns (heart disease, stroke, type 2 diabetes, cancer), to name few. And look in that mirror because you are looking younger.

Here are some tips that I have learned:

1. Rewire your brain that you are no longer hindered by weight.
2. Make friends with your mirror again. You're looking good.
3. Stop avoiding pictures or standing behind the plants.
4. Ditch the big clothes because you worked hard to outgrow them.
5. Don't wear pants that are so large, they fall down in public (yes, it happened to me!).
6. Be prepared for people to hold doors for you, smile, and treat you like you're welcomed in their normally-sized world. It can feel intrusive so prepare yourself.
7. Know that others will be listening to what you're saying, not looking at you because of your weight.
8. Think about how the normally-sized you might upset the social dynamic. You have been the over-sized one in the group forever. How do you fit in now?
9. Realize that the world of travel is not built for fat people. You can now sit comfortably in a middle plane seat, ride on amusement park rides with your family, and can go to any restaurant or theater without crowding others.
10. Be aware that many will never compliment your weight

loss. Don't expect it. It makes people feel weird. Did they approach you to say, "I see you've gained weight?" No, of course not.

11. Depending on your overall size, people generally notice your weight loss once you have parted with about 15 pounds. It varies.

12. For me, people made comments at 30-40 pounds of weight loss.

13. As you approach your goal (like me), you get settled into your new body. Don't be disheartened when the compliments stop. Your self-confidence should not be based on others' validation.

Life on the flip side of obesity is beyond amazing. Not only will you feel better, you will have a renewed enthusiasm for health. While weight loss will not make your life perfect, it will provide you with a healthy and vibrant lifestyle. Pay it forward. Join online weight loss/weight maintenance support groups. Intermittent fasting has numerous Facebook forums which can change your lives. Help others along their journeys.

I am still moving toward maintenance. I am committed to sharing my lessons, challenges, and successes as I move forward. Intermittent fasting is my forever way of living. It is my passion. I have increased my window to 3-4 hours, enjoy increased carbs, and continue to drop pounds as my body experiences added muscle development.

Maintenance as an intermittent faster is real-life. Let's continue to support each other on the journey. May the pure fast be with you. Being timekeepers on our intermittent fasting journeys feels amazing. My very best to all of you! Ready, set,........window is open to amazingly healthy possibilities.

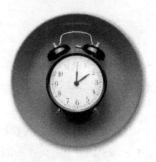

Resources

Articles

Lee, IM, et al. "Physical Activity and Weight Gain Prevention, Women's Health Study." *JAMA.*(2010) March 24; 303 (12) 1173-9.

Volek, J.S, Forsythe, C.E. "The Case for Not Restricting Saturated Fat on Low Carbohydrate Diet." *Nutrition and Metabolism.* 2 (2005) 21.

Westman, E.C., et al., "Effect of 6-month adherence to a very low carbohydrate diet program." *American Journal of Medicine.* 75.5 (2002): 951-953.

Books

Atkins, Robert, M.D. *Dr. Atkins' New Diet Revolution.* 2002.

Avalon, Melanie. *What When Wine: Lose Weight And Feel Great With Paleo-Style Meals, Intermittent Fasting, and Wine.* 2018.

Eisenstein, Charles. *The Yoga of Eating.* 2007.

Fung, Jason. MD. *The Obesity Code Unlocking The Secrets Of Weight Loss.* 2016.

Fung, Jason, MD. *The Diabetes Code Prevent and Reverse Type 2 Diabetes Naturally.* 2018.

Fung, Jason. MD., and Moore Jimmy. *The Complete Guide to Fasting.* 2016.

Herring, Bert, MD. *AC: The Power of Appetite Correction.* 2015.

Herring, Bert, MD. *The Fast-5 Diet And The Fast-5 Lifestyle.* 2015.

McCaffrey, Dee, *The Science of Skinny.* 2012.

Moore, Jimmy and Westman, Eric, MD. *Cholesterol Clarity: What the HDL is Wrong With My Numbers?* 2013.

Moore, Jimmy and Westman, Eric, MD. *Keto Clarity.* 2014.

Phinney, Stephen, MD. and Volek, Jeff, MD. *The Art and Science of Low Carbohydrate Performance Beyond Obesity.* 2012.

Sisson, Mark. *The Keto Reset Diet.* 2017.

Stephens, Gin. *Delay, Don't Deny : Living An Intermittent Fasting Lifestyle.* 2016.

Stephens, Gin. *Feast Without Fear.* 2017.

Taubes, Gary. *Good Calories, Bad Calories: Challenging the Conventional Wisdom on Diet, Weight Control and Disease.* 2011.

Teicholz, Tina. *The Big Fat Surprise: Why Butter, Meat, and Cheese Belong in a Healthy Diet.* 2014.

Westman, Eric, M.D., *A Low Carbohydrate, Ketogenic Diet Manual: No Sugar, No Starch Diet.* 2013.

Blogs, Podcasts, and Other Stuff

2 Keto Dudes Podcast http://2ketodudes.com

Butter Bob Briggs www.buttermakesyourpantsfalloff.com

Delay, Don't Deny Facebook Support Group

(Closed group with membership entry questions).

Dr. Andreas Eenfeldt, The Diet Doctor www.dietdoctor.com

Dr. Eric Berg www.drberg.com

Dr. Mark Hyman http://drhyman.com

Gin Stephens Blog www.ginstephens.com/all-blog-posts

Gin Stephens & Melanie Avalon www.IFpodcast.com

Intensive Dietary Management (IDM) www.idmprogram.com

Nobel Prize www.nytimes.com/2016/10/04/science/yoshinori-ohsumi-nobel-prize-medicine.html

One Meal A Day IF Lifestyle/Facebook Support Group.

(Closed group with membership entry questions).

The Livin La Vida Low-Carb http://www.thelivinlowcarbshow.com

The Obesity Code Podcast. https://obesitycodepodcast.com

Thomas DeLauer. www.thomasdelauer.com

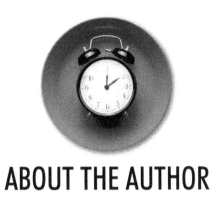

ABOUT THE AUTHOR

Donna Dube is a healthcare consultant and a registered nurse with a Master of Science Degree in Community Health Services Administration, as well as a certification as an Occupational Health Nurse Specialist. Donna has worked for over thirty-five years in health care, and has witnessed the impacts of diabetes, obesity, and unhealthy lifestyles, first-hand. She co-authored an article, "Evaluation of the Impact of the 2012 Rhode Island Health Care Worker Influenza Vaccination Regulations: Implementation Process and Vaccination Coverage, *Journal of Public Health Management and Practice,* 2015.

Donna is a wife, mother, and Nana, who has lost over 100 pounds following an intermittent fasting lifestyle. She has a passion for health and wellness, has studied nutrition at the graduate level, and enjoys coaching others on their paths toward healthier lifestyles.

CPSIA information can be obtained
at www.ICGtesting.com
Printed in the USA
LVHW051831261119
638404LV00003B/97/P